Brain Imbalanced

A Compilation of Research and Autobiography

By S Jenkins, CPA

© 2020 by S Jenkins

All rights reserved. This book or any portion thereof may not be reproduced or used in any manner whatsoever without the express written permission of the publisher except for the use of brief quotations in a book review.

ISBN: 9798729678143

I have tried to recreate events, locales and conversations from my memories of them. In order to maintain their anonymity I have changed the names of individuals and places to protect the privacy of individuals. I also have changed some identifying characteristics and details such as physical properties, occupations and places of residence.

This book is not meant to be used, nor should it be used, to diagnose or treat any medical condition. The contents of this work are not for the purpose of rendering medical advice and are not intended to substitute for professional medical advice, diagnosis or treatment. References are provided for informational purposes only and do not constitute endorsement of any websites or other sources. Readers should be aware that the websites listed in this book may change or disappear between when this work was written and when it is read.

This book is not intended as a substitute for consultation with a licensed practitioner. Please consult with your own physician or healthcare specialist regarding the methodologies mentioned in this book.

For those suffering alone like I have for 40 years...

I hope one day our ailments will be seen by the world as their true nature of being just a chemical imbalance in the brain, synonymous with an insulin deficiency in a diabetic.

I pray for the stigma to end and that there is empathic awareness for those children, adults and seniors struggling with disorders of the mind.

CONTENTS (Charts/Diagrams Herein)

Introduction i

Bipolar Ancestors 1

Phone-Order Bride 7

Reverse Baby Tourism 11

Late-Term Abortion 19

The High-Security Asylum 23

Restraining Orders 27

Predatory Cousins 33

Discovering I Was Bipolar 41

Psychiatric Lockdown Ward 69

Arranged Marriage 87

Postpartum and Fired 99

Hudson and Another Job Lost 125

Fraud Anxiety 151

Manic Unprofessionalism 179

Hopeful Outlook 203

Afterword 233

Introduction

The statistics are staggering; one in five will suffer from a mental illness at some point in their lives. Of the approximately 7.6 billion people on earth today – that means 1.46 billion individuals are, have or will be afflicted by mental illness during some stage of their life; for some all of their lives.

Join Alayna Adams, CPA, on her journey through this book where she scales the bipolar spectrum and has hid her bipolar disorder in corporate America for 20 years. She was able to land job after job successfully, but keeping it was another matter.

Alayna was a head turner in corporate America and at the same time had lost ten jobs and resigned from another two. She was a third generation yet again bipolar in the family.

She had survived childhood incest; those haunting memories followed her for decades and interfered with her relationships with men.

Her bipolar grandfather ended up being murdered, without justice ever served. Her dad was behind bars six times before the doctors realized he had a diagnosis. Both father and son were powerfully wired for domestic violence against their young wives.

She was a Certified Public Accountant, an educated wife, and a mother of two who tried to run the rat race of corporate America and failed at most every turn. Alayna suffered six episodes in her first forty years but amazingly headed off a seventh episode at this seasoned point in life with her acute self-awareness and mastering of medicines in her cabinet.

Her husband, Darrell, would save her from herself time and again. He gave her a lifestyle she had never seen before.

But the brain ailment hounded her. Direly spanked by her mother as a child, she wouldn't do the same to Maddy or Hudson. Had she forgiven her mom? Her mom had wasted away at two jobs and failing health, trying to make ends meet to raise three girls. Her dad didn't want daughters; he had insisted on a son. There were restraining orders, separation filings, and her dad's attempts to break and enter the home. Alayna grew up resenting being born a woman; if anything she could have at least protected her mom better as a son.

Among the multitude of marriage proposals from worthy suitors, Alayna had to hide that she was a mentally unstable party girl who smoked too much.

Alayna's family suffered through many dark times trying to manage her; sometimes hospitalization and the intimidating psychiatric ward were the only avenues.

She made it, though, and never gave up. Her dad had told her about Prime Minister Winston Churchill. Thus she, herself, had resolved if Churchill could live with bipolar disorder and lead his country through World War II, she could do anything as well.

There are roughly 330,000,000 people in the US. That means there are 3.3 million like Alayna who could have bipolar disorder. That gives her hope, anticipation, and some piece of mind that she's not alone. One day when society will overcome its stigma with mental health, and it will eventually as we evolve as a species, she will find the fellow human beings who truly understood her setbacks and fears —her euphoria, episodes, and mistakes. These multitudes of connected individuals dealing with ailments of the brain can be resources to each other on how best to handle work and life events in the future. Life happens. It always does. It doesn't have to be walked alone.

Chapter 1

Bipolar Ancestors

1973

My Dad had bipolar disorder—and was most certainly a severe case at that. He was not diagnosed and treated until his forties, and even then he refused to feel there was anything wrong with him. By then he had shattered his own family and work completely. He was a violent person who refused help. This was learned behavior from his own bipolar father who beat his mother who was thirty years younger.

In his mid-twenties Dad arrived to the port city of Vancouver, which borders the warm Pacific ocean on the western tip of Canada. It is a place where the mountains meet the ocean.

He fought badly with his cousins, who he was staying with temporarily until he found work. His uncle had brought him over from India, and being they were all of Christian decent, everyone wanted to get out of that third world country as a minority; this was a great opportunity to go abroad.

Dad was stubborn, hotheaded, and ill-tempered. He was kicked out by his uncle who didn't tolerate strife between his kids and this unruly new guest.

Dad bounced from one uncle's home to the next until he ended up sitting at the unemployment office for weeks with hopes of landing a job.

No one in the family, in 1973, new that bipolar disorder was even a thing. They did not recognize the scale of symptoms that range from depression to hypermania. Sometimes these symptoms can be of a rapid cycle nature swinging from depression to mania and back to depression within a short time frame. Below is a brief reference chart that can help identify the symptoms to recognize in you or loved ones:

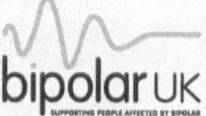

Mood Scale — bipolar UK

This scale is not meant to be definitive but is an indicator of possible behaviours

MANIA	10	Total loss of judgement, exorbitant spending, religious delusions and hallucinations.
	9	Lost touch with reality, incoherent, no sleep, paranoid and vindictive, reckless behaviour.
HYPOMANIA	8	Inflated self-esteem, rapid thoughts and speech, counterproductive simultaneous tasks.
	7	Very productive, everything to excess (phone calls, writing, smoking, tea), charming and talkative.
BALANCED MOOD	6	Self-esteem good, optimistic, sociable and articulate, good decisions and get work done.
	5	Mood in balance, no symptoms of depression or mania. Life is going well and the outlook is good.
	4	Slight withdrawal from social situations, concentration less than usual, slight agitation.
MILD TO MODERATE DEPRESSION	3	Feelings of panic and anxiety, concentration difficult and memory poor, some comfort in routine.
	2	Slow thinking, no appetite, need to be alone, sleep excessive or difficult, everything a struggle.
SEVERE DEPRESSION	1	Feelings of hopelessness and guilt, thoughts of suicide, little movement, impossible to do anything.
	0	Endless suicidal thoughts, no way out, no movement, everything is bleak and it will always be like this.

Call us on 0333 323 3880 | info@bipolaruk.org | bipolaruk.org

— https://www.bipolaruk.org

As related to my Dad, his host families did not recognize any of his moods as atypical behavior. They didn't have any sort of baseline for what normal was for my Dad. The reality was with his arrival, Dad was likely between hypomania and mania. He likely went through significant jet lag arriving to the new world, and coupled with the stimulation and excitement of it, there was likely a lack of sleep, which all this could trigger manic behavior.

His critical goal was to get a job and eventually sponsor his own family of five younger siblings, a mother, and a father. He tried finding work on his own but then finally sat at an unemployment office for weeks until the secretary irately said to her boss, "You need to get this guy a job. He makes puppy eyes at me all day. He's been here for weeks, sir!" My Dad would retell this story amusingly in later years.

Dad had only partly finished school in his home country where he wanted to be a poet and writer and teach English. But in typical Eastern fashion, his dad, also bipolar and very much untreated, pushed him into STEM subjects (science, technology, engineering, and math). He needed to make money, not be an unemployed writer.

Grandpa wanted Dad to be an engineer and pushed him into that field of study. The sad irony is my dad would have done really well as a writer. He was Shakespearean in his bipolar ability of rhyming couplets; the manic energy would surge into euphoric writing. Dad would write beautiful poetry effortlessly.

But here Dad was now, far from being a writer. He was sent to Fort McMurray's nickel mine, close to the Arctic Circle line, and then later to work on the railroads as hard manual labor. For immigrants there wasn't much to choose from in those years – those decades when racial barriers and fears strongly eclipsed most employers' hiring decisions; the locals didn't want to hire a person of color — it was a risk.

Racial divides were strong back then even if one wasn't black. In Vancouver during the 1970s there was a phone number to call, which I heard of later that my uncles spoke of, where if you were pushed around by white folks, a brown person could call, and there were young brown men waiting by that corded rotary dial phone. They were waiting with bats and ready to jump in their long trunk cars and head to the rescue. Like those awesome cars in *The Dukes of Hazard*.

They were an informal dispatch service, because the police weren't going to help a brown boy get out of trouble. It was like being the black people in the US. In Canada brown people were the underclass. They wouldn't call the police out of practical purposes; the law enforcement would not effectively help. They would call their fellow brown brothers.

Dad learned the hard way from the men he worked alongside on the railroad. One railroad worker Dad bunked with, saw Dad removing socks when he felt his feet had frozen, and the coworker corrected him, "Paul, don't double your socks when you go out; that's worse for circulation. Your foot will freeze off." He shared a small cabin with another immigrant, and the only bright part was receiving a picture of my mom from abroad—the girl he was going to marry. He'd kiss that picture he admitted decades later, he was so enamored with her.

He once told me the conversation he had with an aged Indian man from his time up north, who had told him, "Son, don't marry white. Bring your own bride from overseas; never marry white. Bring an Indian girl here. You won't mesh here with these people. You'll be unhappy." There was discrimination both ways back then; older generations looked at different skin colors with distrust and fear.

Dad had the pressure of sponsoring a family of five siblings back in the subcontinent. My paternal grandfather had given his life savings to send him to college, which Dad failed miserably at.

Midway through college, when word came from Canada that Dad's paperwork was ready, Grandpa sent him abroad with many hopes for Dad to sponsor him, his mom, and siblings to the new land. Grandpa would die before he ever got the chance to see North America and its glory, beauty, and organized society.

Dad really had to bear the intermediate brunt of change to make it markedly better for his future offspring and generations to come. Otherwise we would be living in rural India in the small village Grandpa raised his family in. It is likely the conditions may have become only incrementally better with each passing generation if the family had stayed and not migrated. But Grandpa and Dad worked together to break this cycle of rural living.

My father had spent fifteen dollars during his layover in Japan on a haircut and food, which he direly regretted later when getting to the mainland of British Columbia (BC), the western most province in the country of Canada.

He arrived to the new country with only a remainder twenty dollars. This was a lot of money back then, but he had spent almost half of it in Japan, thinking maybe he was getting a good deal on a haircut and a nice meal. He had no idea about foreign exchange translations. He certainly also had no idea about predatory airport pricing.

My Dad still cries to this day at times about never being able to see his dad before Grandpa died and never being able to avenge Grandpa's murder. My Dad was behaviorally oppositional and stubborn toward his father in childhood — perhaps these were the early manifestations of bipolar tendencies or just a difficult father-son relationship with both having untreated brain imbalances. Grandpa was speculated to have bipolar disorder as well given many hallmark symptoms of extreme anger and mood swings.

Grandpa had died tragically and mysteriously. His death was murder but was unofficially announced as food poisoning. There was no autopsy done. But the onlookers at the funeral realized the reality and talked about the incident. He was murdered in the late 1970s right before I was born.

My grandfather was an accountant in India, a general accountant who did the village records. He needed money as he was to come abroad and had land he could sell that was jointly owned by his other siblings.

He had traveled to another town where his siblings resided, the inheritance was to be settled and his part of it cashed so that he had enough money to travel abroad and settle the rest of his family in the new country. Grandpa stayed at his sister's house the night before he died, and the sister's sons allegedly had poisoned his breakfast before the settlement could happen and buyout be given to him.

When my grandfather's body arrived, it was said that his lips were black. The sister's family had announced he had had a heart attack and to bury the body quickly.

They likely were scared that Paul would come back from abroad, the oldest son, who wasn't juvenile like the other harmless brothers still in India. He would come back and ask questions, or worse. He was known to have anger issues already. Dad was known to break things when mad.

My mom's dad, Samuel, attended the funeral. He was there as this was his daughter's father-in-law after all. Samuel also had deemed it was poison, quietly.

It clearly was not a heart attack as the people who hosted him the recent evening had said. With Grandpa out of the way, there was more inheritance for this sister and her sons.

They didn't pass anything along to Dad's family. Grandpa was not the favorite of his family for the reason that he'd converted to Christianity. That inheritance money allocated to him would have helped the financial situation of Dad's rural family and funding their new life abroad.

My dad never gained closure; he wanted to go back and avenge his father's death. If you didn't have a lot of money, forget bringing the cops in. They wouldn't do anything for the lower middle class; such cases weren't taken seriously. The system was corrupt.

But Dad had to worry about his five siblings and bringing his widowed mother over to the new country. He had to focus on work. There wasn't enough money to buy a ticket back.

Chapter 2

Phone-Order Bride

1975

Dad sponsored my mom two years after he arrived to the New World. It was an arranged marriage committed to over the phone between both my grandfathers.

The bride and groom only saw pictures of each other. In India, Mom had no wedding, just a small celebratory send-off where she got dressed up and her family took a handful of solo pictures of her. The families did a groom-less party and sent her off with prayers, jewelry, and clothing.

Mom met Dad at the airport for the very first time. She washed her own wedding dishes after the party that was put on by the couple for the relatives, and she washed those dishes all throughout the night. They couldn't afford a restaurant, so she cooked her own wedding meal—and cleaned. Everyone was an in-law; they neither jumped in to help her nor did she ever venture to ask for their help.

Dad had hit Mom on the third night after their wedding night. She was shaken. Men hit women in India—but so soon? That was a bad sign. She hid the abuse from her family and seven siblings for years with the exception of her brother, Christopher, who was already living in Europe and studying for the Chartered Accountant (CA) exam. Christopher kept insisting to Mom, even after her first child was born to this man, that she should leave him. Christopher often insisted, "I'll send a ticket. Bring your child or leave her with her father; just leave him today."

But Mom stayed in the marriage with the faulty notion that the kid needed her father. Also she could never imagine abandoning her daughter to her mother-in-law and husband. The true marital reality of Christopher's sister at nineteen years of age married to a man who was violent was kept hidden. Back then bipolar disorder was virtually unknown, and everyone thought Dad just had anger issues. Dad's family fudged a lot of facts at the marriage proposal time; one example was they said he was an engineer. He hadn't even finished his second year of college.

He was nine years Mom's senior, but they told her family it was a difference of six. In fact Dad's paperwork was made in his teen years and he was shown to be born two years younger since he'd repeated grade five twice. My grandfather thought it best to dial back his age in paperwork. This seemingly benign but ill-thought-out action would table Dad's retirement benefits that he badly needed after walking the streets alone for twenty-five years. The help from the government didn't start until he was sixty-seven, not sixty-five, in actuality. Such decisions to adjust birthdays are often made in the South Asian subcontinent, partly because it's unknown; a Grandma might have kept track of what season a baby was born. Then gauge roughly against the crop rotations or harvests peg a week, and then narrow down to an arbitrary day of the week. In this fashion you arrive at a birthday. This over simplified approach has ramifications decades later.

At least nine years of an age difference between my parents was still a big improvement from my paternal grandparents' age difference. My Grandpa married Grandma when she was fifteen and he was forty-five. He was born in 1910. He was a widower and had married again. Back then fifteen was not a rare age for especially rural men and women to get married.

So all things considered my maternal grandparents thought it was a steady prospect with financial security for their daughter at the time and took Dad's family's word. Their daughter would go abroad to a land of awe, inspiration, and sophistication. It would be amazing for her.

There was no social media or anything as such to do a snooping dig and verification of a suitor. There was no Internet to tap into back then, where you can Google a name and find some digital footprint or commonality of mutual connections to corroborate with.

There was also no foresight to engage in private investigators, just faith in that it's a good family from what you have heard through the community network. Parents typically would say a prayer for their daughters and hope for the best. In typical Eastern thinking, the parents of the groom felt if he got married, his issues like anger will remedy themselves. They figured there would be kids eventually, and he would outgrow his stubborn anger and shake off his frequent temper if he bonded with someone and had the responsibilities of a family. The parents of the bride were told the groom had a good job abroad, which is always important in these cases as he's going to be the sole breadwinner.

My mom knew very little English. What she did learn in the next few years was from watching daytime soap operas while her husband was out. She only had an eighth grade education from India, from a village school. English was just one subject; the rest was all in a foreign tongue.

Mom loved fashion—books, not so much.

She was a great cook. She loved domestic responsibilities and excelled in this area compared to her sisters; they joked she loved to eat and make things all the time. She was the perfect Indian wife of those times. Tragically that's all my dad ever complimented – the culinary skills. Mom would lay his socks, underwear, and clothes out for him, her friends telling her, "You're spoiling him." Maybe she thought his anger would cool if she served him to the highest degree.

My parents first born came along ten months after they married. My older sister Delilah's infancy was a turbulent one. My father tried to strangle Delilah while in her crib during a fight where Dad's mother Edna and my mom ran to rescue Delilah. Dad was raging over some trivial family dispute and targeted Delilah as the cause. He'd break dishes at times in anger, and my mom would clean it up, tears streaming down her face that she hid; that might set him off again—the tears.

My mom lived in a crowded one bedroom apartment in downtown Vancouver with Edna and Dad's five younger siblings, all unmarried and still at home. Some of them yet were to come of age. One of her sisters-in-law had a vendetta against Mom. Likely this was a product of some sort of naive jealousy that crept in upon having to share her older brother's attention with another woman suddenly.

This sister once told my dad when he walked in from work that Mom was on the phone with her 'lover'. My Dad stopped her in her tracks and slapped his sister across the face. That time my mom was spared, but tensions ran high, and usually Mom was the one to take the beating.

Chapter 3

Reverse Baby Tourism

1979

I was born in the late 1970s when my mom went to India and had me there. It was too difficult to take his abuse and be pregnant with a toddler in tow at the same time; she needed her family's help. I was born in India, in a small town. Mom spent most of her time in a rural village where her father was the town mayor, but to give birth, she went to a relatively bigger center.

Mom's first child was a cesarean section. However I turned out to be a natural birth. She was in dire pain and told the doctor to do another C-section, but he refused, and she had the most painful V-back (a vaginal delivery after a C-section). You risk the rupturing of the uterus with a V-back. No future kids can be born of that ruptured womb.

It's a blessing in disguise, though, not to have an operation abroad. Even to this day, sanitary conditions are not nearly the same as compared to North America's hospitals and medical expertise. People die of infection from knee replacements these days while in a sub-standard hospital in the subcontinent. A C-section in the 70s would have been risky.

It was baby tourism in reverse, where most come to North America for an opportune baby delivery and grab citizenship for the newborn and fly back. Some shamefully even start benefits in Canada and fly back and continue to collect from a blind government while they have riches from factories, businesses, or land they own overseas. It is truly gluttonous behavior.

My mom had to go the opposite way for her protection. The family was already settled in Canada, a first world country, a world power and valuable birthplace with automatic citizenship. But ironically I was born in a third world country out of the safety necessity for Mom. The fact that I was not born on Canadian soil later proved to be a major issue. I had my Canadian citizenship revoked when I was in my forties, this was a sad situation of my Dad erroneously being given his citizenship by the Canadian Government in the 1970s as they had overlooked he had been in a hit and run accident that he had left the scene of which meant his citizenship application should have been rejected and tabled till a few years later upon a re-application. His citizenship that was awarded to him in error nullified my citizenship four decades later after I had lived in Canada for twenty two years, paid taxes, and renewed my passport multiple times. I had acquired my citizenship because of his citizenship, which now was discovered to be issued on faulty grounds. It was very frustrating that the government decided to eject my citizenship based on a dig of his records. Had I been born in Canada, like my older sister and younger sister, there wouldn't have been any questions or revocations. I would have been born on Canadian soil like them and the status couldn't be taken away. But despite the fact that Mom had me in India I am deeply grateful for her safety and sanity that was made possibly only by taking refuge with her family in her home country during that pregnancy and delivery time.

Reflecting back to my birth time, when Dad heard over the phone from Mom it was a girl again, he was broken and said, "Just stay there; I don't need you all to come back." He wanted boys, not girls. All she was giving him was girls. She was gravely saddened; he was just like the rest of the men in that regard too. India had and still has a strong angle against female births. Girls are a liability, boys are an asset. To get her married, to pay for all that, to be dishonored if she is raped or pregnant without marriage, a million things fly through parents' minds on the horrible what-ifs. She can't work in the fields as well as a boy can. They have to pay for two pieces of clothing for her versus one for a boy; that is how the very bottom of the rung feels in India. And some of these fears trickle upward to other societal classes like the one Dad and Edna were born in. Both mother and son weren't happy at the fact Mom kept bearing girls and expressed it to her at one point or another.

Following my birth, Mom rushed back to save her marriage. I was in the care of my maternal Grandma, whom they said died of the guilt and pain of arranging her daughter to a man like this; finally it was uncovered the misfortune and difficult circumstances her daughter weathered for years. My Grandma had died shortly after I was born; she had taken care of me a few months right before her demise. They said I cried when she died and kept watching for her from my crib, and when they would call her name, I'd temporarily stop crying.

I came to Canada in the first ten months of my life. In the early 1980s, we shifted to a small mining town in northern BC, away from Dad's siblings who were still in the bustling port city. The copper mine was hiring anyone who wanted to work four days off and four days on with twelve-hour shifts daily. Workers would need to take a two-hour ride to the open-pit mine further north in the Cascadian mountain area.

In this town the sun went down around 3:00 p.m. in the winters, a depressing and engulfing darkness which may have been an exacerbating situation for someone with bipolar disorder who remained untreated. Conversely the sun set at 11:00 p.m. in the summers, which would induce insomnia and create a manic situation.

The dark years would continue for my mom and spread to what seemed like an eternity. Mom had considered ending her life at one point, and not just her own.

I remember this story as though I had clear cognition at the time but I was an infant only at that time – so vividly can I understand the emotion and circumstances. My mom had driven the car down to the lake. She was alone with my father who kept beating her. At the time, Delilah was five, and I was two. Delilah was confused why Mom had gotten out onto the lake's beach without us. My mom stood and pondered a while; she had made up her mind to drive the car into the lake, with all of us in it. End it, end the misery – her emotions told her. But then she started to cry, and maybe the faith, maybe the hope, maybe some slight breeze from God told her, "Don't do it, don't end your children's lives. Don't end your life, it's a sin." Go back, she was being told, in the fiber of her being. Something must have held her. Something told her to not make the emotional decision that is irreversible once acted upon. Such decisions are not temporary, but are permanent. The impulsivity didn't take over Mom completely.

Mom went back to that house of horrors. She stayed with Dad for sixteen years, because the girls would need a father. She felt the kids needed both their parents; and had convinced herself that she should stay in it for the kids. This is a classic mistake because if the kids see the abuse, that is worse. Witnessing dysfunctional and abusive relationships affects children's own future relationships detrimentally more times then not. A stressed mom or dad isn't a good parent. Life is tough single, but it's not a pressure cooker of emotional, physical, verbal and/or sexual abuse as otherwise may be in a troubled marital relationship.

My mom tarried for years, and the societal thought plagued her: Who will marry a divorcée's daughters? It's hard enough getting daughters married. You have to wait and pray for a good proposal. What if I ever leave? Uncle Christopher had offered over and over again to send her the means to escape. The Eastern societal pressures can be a meat grinder for women to stay in relationships, and specifically more so in the old country where there is no financial independence for a divorced woman other then living with her parents if they are still alive and accept her. Ironically Mom could have left without financial worry as she was in Canada but sadly didn't know about benefits available or that the concept of women's shelters existed to be able to escape quickly.

Thankfully my mom had one Indian friend in the mining town who gave her some consolation. This was a lady who understood her culture, marital pain, and anguish; she was a lady with children and the same value system and ethnicity, and her husband was good to her. My mom was in awe at their healthy relationship and yearned for one like that herself.

This lady helped Mom secretly get her citizenship in 1985 through the mail – a fact hidden from my dad. They still keep in touch, my mom and her. This friend has lost a son to drunk driving. To outlive a child is the worst thing to happen to a parent. I'll always remember this friend as Mom's lifeline.

In the mining town as I grew older I was more adamant to be vocal and protect Mom as I realized at some point Dad never hit us, he only hit Mom. So I was confident I could be a sort of shield of hers. An example of this is one time I had to get in the middle of Dad and Mom, as he had held a crystal bowl decoration piece, a big one, over Mom's head to hit her with it. Dad was on the way to the mine's bus stop up the street that morning, the mine's bus would pick up miners in the same neighborhood and continue the route through town. He couldn't be late, but Mom was on the phone earlier with Uncle Christopher, and something had switched Dad's mood. He was in his blue and black checkered flannel shirt that would usually smell like the mine when he came home. I was eating breakfast before school and jumped out of my chair. I remember it like it was yesterday, a vividly bad memory etched in my mind forever.

My mom hit me quite a bit in those years when still living with Dad; I was the act-up kind of kid. My grandfather Samuel had once said to Mom that I wasn't normal; and she was concerned also. Under her own tremendous pressures, she was short tempered with me, I was never on the straight and narrow like my sister Delilah. Her temper was understandable to me in hindsight, living in that pressure cooker environment.

When I had kids, I told myself I would not hit. Just spank, no back of the hand or wooden ladle. I was smacked with the wooden ladle once for going to a friend's house without telling Mom. I had dark-blue bruise marks all over my back. My father actually talked to my mother about her severe reaction that time. I had slipped away to a Mexican girlfriend's house; Mom had told me specifically I couldn't go to her house. Mom and her generation had their own fears of the unknown. White people were only somewhat trustworthy in her mind, and other non-Indian races were to be entirely mistrusted and feared. We weren't to go to any friends' houses unless both sisters were invited; she was worried about harm. She never suspected her family of possible wrong doing but strangers, yes. Sexual assault mainly happens from people you know, not strangers. Sadly she never realized where the true threat was but she would later in life.

After that horribly bruising beating, I didn't want to change in front of the girls in the locker room at school during gym class because I was worried child services would take me away if the girls noticed and reported the excessive marks on my back. That was grade five. I loved my family; that's all I knew. And when I became a mom, myself, I understood and was in awe how my mom did all of it alone and weathered life solely. I never held it against her, all those slaps and that one horrible beating. For when you become a mom yourself you start to understand the gravity of the tremendous responsibility and stressors that come with motherhood.

Much later in life I reflected on a particular call from her on this subject in my mid-thirties, and the conversation was a tearful one on her end. She was crying, "Alayna, please forgive me. I hit you a lot; I regret that." I laughed it off. I never thought it was even a thing until she said it. I later realized she was going through a bout of depression. Even in her older years, she missed her by then X-husband somewhat and sometimes would say she would rather have a house with him in it versus an empty house with just her sitting there. I would take those slaps again, the loneliness is worse she'd say decades later.

Chapter 4

Late-Term Abortion

1986

Our family would drive down to Vancouver from the mining town almost every weekend. Dad's family was still settled there. Grandma Edna was living with her other two sons who were now both married to women they sponsored from overseas, and they lived in a squalling joint-family system. I speculate it is an economic need that does that, not a desire to live together. One roof is cheaper—one rent.

It was an eight-hour drive at forty-five to sixty kilometers per hour, winding through slow mountain turns with a deep gorge and raging white waters below. Look away for an instant, and that cement block around the turn might not keep your car on the road. No air bags then so likely you'd be dead on the rocks. Your car might blow up.

We had a Pontiac hatchback, and my dad would sometimes put me in his lap when he drove. It was the most exhilarating feeling to help hold the steering wheel. I was also allowed to sit in the trunk and wobble around, but one time my head hit the side because my mom slipped off the highway into the ditch in icy weather. There were certainly some precarious rides. We lived in a mountainous area and those mountains and scenery stay with me to this day.

We had some good moments during childhood in that valley town. There were the trips to McDonalds; Dad would take us and we felt elated. Mom would never do that. In actuality I am guessing she was scared to touch the pocketbook, because he might fly off the handle. He liked spoiling us girls. As kids we had some happy times. But Delilah was three years older and understood the marital abuse going on. She was chronically constipated and had eczema, which only cleared up once Mom left Dad.

My younger sister, Emilia, was born near the end of the 1980s. While Mom was pregnant, my dad made phone calls like a madman trying to figure out how to arrange a late term abortion. Maybe he would need to take Mom to the US. The local clinics refused because the grounds for the abortion he stated were "It's a girl."

A dream saved my little sister's life; my father would tell it himself later. In the dream he was shouting at a kitten in order to intimidate her to get off the bed, and the kitten looked on at him, completely benign and innocent. God was angry with him, right then and there, he felt it. God was furious because he had waved his hand and been very loud towards this scared, helpless, tiny kitten. That was the extent of his dream. He hadn't heard a voice, but the feeling of disappointment and shaking anger came from somewhere. Dad awoke with a new outlook. He told Mom, "No, I must not kill this child. God would be angry."

Mom was already at the threshold of knowing the child's soul, as it was already beyond the first trimester. The first trimester is one that is beheld by some cultures as one in which the child is without soul, and only a piece of flesh. It was too late anyways for an abortion she knew. It would be wrong. And it was killing her to know her daughter would go to waste in some medical laboratory.

Dad already tried strangling Delilah and shunning Alayna overseas, but fate intervened with Emilia. Fate thwarted his plans. The daughter was allowed to be born, but my mom went to the hospital three months early and admitted there. She was flown from the mining town to the lower mainland's hospital.

Emilia was born very premature and less than four pounds. My mom's blood pressure was very high throughout the pregnancy. She was so stressed; each girl was lighter than the last. Her sister, Jennifer, had come from overseas to help with the household in the meantime. Aunt Jennifer was a second mom to us. She was so wise in her ways. Aunt Jennifer hadn't had any biological children of her own.

Mom and Aunt Jennifer had a traditional Indian upbringing where domestic tasks were encouraged and the focus was to one day marry and raise a family successfully. My mom was the baby of the family they would say, although not the youngest. She was favored – she loved to cook luxuriously for everyone and demonstrated her affection for her family in that manner. Her dad had always treated her mom with respect and kindness. Mom had grown up in a very different environment, in a healthy way, unlike Dad's childhood where he witnessed his mom being beaten by his dad, and frequently.

Grandpa Samuel was torn one time as he left his daughter at the airport and flew back overseas… Mom had cried on his shoulder for a while. He knew how bad it was for her and encouraged her to leave Dad but she was committed to the relationship because of her feeling of obligation to her children and keeping the family together.

Grandpa Samuel died of blood cancer a few years after Emilia was born. He had been a heavy smoker, especially in the entire last decade of his life when he no longer had Grandma by his side. Grandma had always told Grandpa during their many years together that she wanted to be first to go as she couldn't bear the loss of him.

Chapter 5

The High-Security Asylum

1988

As the seasons changed, so did Dad's moods; my mom anticipated it early. He was never bad to the kids, but Mom bore the brunt of it. She would walk on eggshells not to say anything. Even the slightest thing would set him off, and the verbal and physical abuse was there.

Near the time of our escape out of that mining town home, Dad started turning a bit on Delilah and me. I remember I closed the fridge door too hard, and he jumped out of his skin and ripped into me verbally, running in from the adjacent room. That wasn't normal for our dad. He would literally froth at the mouth. My mom had never seen anything like it. Spittle stuck to the lips, white spittle—not transparent— when he was seething mad and yelling.

One year Mom went to the hospital, and the emergency room staff had said, "No, you couldn't have fallen in the tub." She insisted, yes, she did. A bleeding ear? She didn't want to incriminate her husband. How would she survive without him? He didn't let her get her citizenship; recall she had acquired that secretively from him through mailing from a friend's house in the mid-1980s. She had no idea of benefits in a country that is more than giving to those in need. She couldn't survive on her own she felt.

In the next few years before the 1990s, there was growing knowledge of mental illness at least in the medical community. The mine doctor suspected Dad was struggling with something of the sort, and the doctor called the emergency contact, my mom, and told her that her husband was unstable. He had erratic behavior and anger towards fellow miners and it seemed to be on a downward trajectory. But he had had some good years at the mine in the beginning. Dad had been given multiple promotions before the erratic behavior started, but he had said it's too lonely at the top; and further into his mining career the instability of bipolar disorder was showing at work too, not just home. My mom was frustrated with Dad's passing up of promotions earlier in his career. That would have been money and prestige in the local community of brown people—her husband, a mine foreman.

Dad wasn't keeping his moody conflicts at home anymore. As the illness remained untreated, it ebbed into his work life too. Work was starting to suffer and become jeopardized after working in the mine for over ten years.

He refused to take medicines. As with this illness, there is that grandiose feeling when episodic—there is nothing wrong with me, it's a conspiracy, it's the rest of the world. The so-called diagnosis is a moneymaking scam of the pharmacies and that's all it is… many delusional thoughts float through your impulsive mind during an episode, reasons that seem completely logical to you at the time.

Mom would slip the doctor's prescribed medicines into Dad's warm milk at night. But he was starting to go through a depression of sorts as the medicines caused excessive sleep and brought his mania down in a nose dive. During mania he would read the Bible all throughout the night and memorize entire pages of verses only to repeat them verbatim to Mom. He was sleepless originally, then these medicines started. His original manic stage transpired into depression and finding a balance was difficult. Patients sometimes discontinue medicines as they feel worse on them. They are no longer euphoric in mania, but lethargic and slowed down due to anti-psychotic drugs. It takes a trial and error process of modifying medicines and a willingness on the part of the patient to participate. So Dad's ride of the sinusoidal curve continued for a long period of time. Riding the ups and downs of that curve, the up being mania and the low being depression with just a small amount of time at the balanced middle. The anti-psychotic medicines bring you down, sometimes far too down, and then you bounce up later but slowly.

Dad went overseas after starting treatment, a trip to find a second wife so she could bear him a son, as then it was not known that the gender of a child is determined by the father, not the mother. As a spouse you find your mind, body, and soul equal in your other half. Why then have a second spouse? Polygamy is forbidden in the New World, and in the Old World, many religions don't allow it, but Dad bent the rules based on his raging mind.

Mom's family, who hosted him in India, dissuaded him from the subject, and he came back further clinically depressed and unsuccessful at getting married a second time. Part of them wanted to avenge Mom's suffering at his hands over the years and they were considering admitting him involuntarily to the asylum in India where the inpatients are covered in lice and fleas. But their sister had three daughters, and he was the sole breadwinner. So they considered the pragmatic side. With three girls Mom likely couldn't get married again – it would be a rarity if a worthy suitor proposed to her. Finally Dad was sent back on his return ticket, as this unstable and somewhat now-medicated man was the only future chance their sister may have at a somewhat financially decent life.

The mine let Dad work an easier job, but he had a difficult time staying on his medications. When he started to feel better he figured he didn't need them anymore. He didn't understand fully that it is a permanent condition that needs sustained medicines to circulate in one's system for life.

During these years Dad was up and down. Additionally the mine went on strike so he became a cab driver and we moved to the lower mainland so he could start to work there. It was still a roller coaster, Dad would have run-ins with law enforcement as they were dispatched to break up his fist fights with strangers and people he knew. He was erratic again. One time when the cops put him before the judge, Dad started swearing female vulgarities at the lady judge and the court quickly realized he was mentally unstable and she immediately ordered him to the high security asylum for assessment and care. We visited him there once as a family, Mom, my sisters and me. Dad was in a post-manic phase, extremely medicated and also extremely depressed. He ran from the visitation room ashamed and crying after exchanging the first few greeting sentences with us. Emilia was only a toddler then, and intimidated by the surroundings that looked like a jail. It was an asylum down by the river with a view of the industrious river that had cargo boats and logs floating by. The windows I looked through didn't face the mountains. It was a cold, clammy, jail-like institutional building solely lit by cold white fluorescent tube lighting. We were sad to see him in that state but no one wanted to take him home permanently, we were too scared of his rage. The mine opened back up later and we discontinued our rental in the lower mainland and moved back into our vacant home in the mining town so Dad could resume work. Mom was remorseful while Dad was at a low point and needed her. Perhaps the medications would be a consistent part of his future she hoped and life would stabilize. But she didn't realize that upon his upswing from depression he would digress into his baseline behaviors again.

Chapter 6

Restraining Orders

1990

In an effort to escape finally, Mom convinced Dad that she wanted to visit her youngest brother a few provinces over during the summer, with the girls while Dad continued working. She did not disclose she had no intent to come back to him.

My mom had saved $5,000, a huge amount in the 80s, before leaving him. She was going to take it on the trip back east when she'd escape to her brother's house. This money was slowly collected from grocery change; it took her a decade to gather the sum. She had opened her own secret account. That was her runaway stash. But during a random fight, she used it as arson— a naive mistake to uncover the means she had to leave and have a more comfortable start to a new life. He demanded for her to authorize he take the funds. He took her to the bank the same day.

That summer when Delilah was thirteen, I was age ten and Emilia was age three, the four of us went to the prairies to 'visit' her youngest brother, who was still single. It was not intended to be a temporary visit, but a permanent move. We ended up living there for a year. We all lived together in a small apartment, in a congested manner —my mom and her sister, Jennifer, who had also immigrated during Emilia's birth. Aunt Jennifer had sponsored her own family that also joined the congestion. Aunt

Jennifer and Mom worked the fast-food restaurant that their brother owned.

Delilah and I did middle school there. Delilah was markedly older than most other kids in her class. My mom unfairly held Delilah back in grade one, as she felt she wasn't skilled and confident enough. This was a poor decision; Mom didn't consider the embarrassment and setback Delilah would feel. The teachers discouraged Mom from holding her back; they said she'd catch up and do fine in grade two. So although Delilah was there years older than me she was only one grade my senior.

In Manitoba, the schools never closed until it was –33°C, and the wind-chill factor was officially ignored, it could be –40°C with wind chill but schools were still kept open. This was very frustrating. Unless the official temperature was on or below –33°C, you had to go to school. We weren't used to the prairie winds. The mining town was sandwiched in the middle of a valley; although it would snow, it wasn't as dry. It wasn't as windy. But in this new part of the country it was biting cold. If you lived close enough to the school, you walked; the bus was reserved for those very far away, and most had to pay a fee for it.

Delilah's and my eyelashes would freeze in the winter air, and we had scant gear. We were a stark contrast to the white locals who had adapted and would ski and enjoy the elements. The majority of immigrant parents didn't know about the proper gear as they came from the tropics. Back then you'd look at other schoolmates with wonder, they seemed much more comfortable in the subzero temperatures. This walk to school of five minutes seemed like two hours in the frigid temperatures to us.

It wasn't thriftiness on my mom's part that precluded us from good winter gear. It was the lack of knowledge on what was out there, as an immigrant family from the tropics. The Western fashion knowledge wasn't one my mom knew about either. How my sister and I wished she'd pick up a magazine and plan our clothing. We never had magazines and couldn't imagine spending the money on them. We had no idea what fashion was. The other kids looked cool. They had friends. We didn't.

It may have helped for us to dress at least somewhat like the kids at school. My mom would buy the same outfits for Delilah and me from *Army & Navy* or *Sears*. These outfits were ugly—so ugly—floral patterns mostly. What made sense in India for fashion she figured would work here—a mix of floral patterns. We did a lot of corduroy also. It didn't help us with the friend situation at school.

On the prairies there was a different kind of racism in school. They hated the local red Indians, as they called them, and they mistook us for them. This mix up in ethnicity actually happened in the mining town too at times. It was a rough sixth grade on the prairies, but also the mining town had the same racial divides. I had only one friend in grade two, but one day she said "My mom said I can't play with you because you are a Red Indian." It was so hurtful, not to mention completely inaccurate as well. Dots versus feathers; they never understood which one we were.

On the prairies, there were no mountains or ocean, just flat terrain every which way you looked. The cold would cut you to the bone on this landscape. We were many hundreds of miles beyond North Dakota's northern border, far up in Canada but still not north of 60 degrees latitude where the Arctic Circle starts. Winter temperatures here would go as low as $-55°C$. Sometimes you could see a white aurora in the sky – the northern lights. These lights were not in the full radiant electrifying colors seen further north in Alaska or Scandinavia; what I saw were just white waves in a black sky above. Nonetheless the lights were both beautiful and haunting at the same time, making you stop and look for a while – almost in a hypnotizing way.

In this prairie town there were mosquito summers and cold, windy, dry winters. In one of the two summers we lived there, city trucks were dispatched to drive up and down the streets to spray mosquito deterrent. It had rained heavily and the layers of larvae underground came up in abundance, mosquitoes were horrifically everywhere.

Meanwhile, Dad had sold everything in the house when Mom said she was never coming back. His mania was acutely worse now. Before leaving she had given up and couldn't convince him to take medicines daily. Without her, his bipolar mania would not give him any chance of rational thought where he would be propelled to go back onto his medications. Such medications that were ironically within reach in the kitchen medicine cabinet. In his mania, he sold the new electric-blue car we had bought as a family to cousins for pennies on the dollar, and they shortchanged him on it quite a bit, but he was episodic, euphoric and didn't think twice about even negotiating it. Dad then bought a minivan and drove to Alaska where he hit a moose that was monopolizing the street, totaling the van. Dad was originally headed back to Vancouver from a daytrip in Seattle, where he had picked up a hitchhiker on the way back. When Dad had asked where he was going, this young hippy gentleman told Dad he was going to Alaska and would continue to hitchhike up the Alaskan Highway until he made it there. My father's thoughts were rushing, the wheels turning too quickly in his manic unharnessed mind and he decided to drive this stranger all the way to Alaska based on a split second impulsive decision.

In Alaska, Dad had a thirty-two-ounce steak, which he threw up on the side of the road after leaving the restaurant and driving in his van a short while; he would laugh at that memory later. He had spent all his money earned from the sale of his preciously accumulated home goods, on gaudy Alaskan souvenirs instead, and a lot of them. These buying sprees are common for a manic mind. I could live without seeing another Alaskan logo-etched glass for the rest of my life. He had given them to us as gifts later.

While we lived on the prairies, Dad would leave threatening messages for Mom on the answering machine which held cassette tapes and recorded everything. He was desperate to have his family back and still lived on the West Coast while we lived 1,400-plus miles east of him. The separation lawyer my mom had engaged by then had advised my mom to get the answering machine and she was to keep the cassette tapes for evidence later. It was upsetting to hear the phone messages at all hours; there was a time difference, and bipolar disorder keeps you up all night with no sleep when manic. Dad was awake around the clock with manic energy in his voice.

The lawyer also told Mom to buy a gun. Mom never did, she couldn't even think of owning a gun. She didn't know how to shoot. Mom didn't even know that shooting lessons existed, and those would have cost money anyways. Money she needed to feed her kids with instead. So she filed a restraining order as protection.

Dad drove for three days to our apartment from Vancouver, crossing province after province. He had brought those souvenirs from his recent Alaskan trip in paper bags with our names and attributes on them, penned in black thick marker. Even for Mom, there was something written in our foreign language, not derogatory but meant to appease.

The police were called by Mom when Dad arrived. He had rung the apartment buzzer as the main door to enter the lobby was always locked and he didn't have the patience to shoulder surf in. We were all scared and nervous; he had left so many threatening messages. We were all standing in the apartment complex's front yard, the world watching. Dad begged the police to let him take us on a trip and Mom to come along as a "servant," as he said it in his native tongue, and that he wouldn't touch her body. It was a very exposing conversation and experience, as a family to hear it, his pleas, all together in front of officers. It was a very naked, awkward, and embarrassing experience.

The police drove Dad all the way back to the western most province lines making sure he was sent back to the border given the restraining order in place. He returned to Vancouver with his tears shedding for days, driving back alone. He was so desperate he agreed to Mom's conditions on a later phone call. Dad would sign the house over to Mom, so she would have her own financial assets and have resources.

Recall, the only way we had escaped from there earlier was that we went on an alleged family vacation to visit Mom's youngest brother, but Mom had intended we weren't going back. I was the one who begged her at age ten to go back. I wanted my old house back; the apartment was congested. A two-bedroom apartment with eight people in it. Recall by then Aunt Jennifer's family from India, consisting of her husband and adopted son, had come to stay after she successfully sponsored them – compounding the number in the apartment.

A year of school had gone by, and the next summer I was dying to go home. I didn't really miss Dad, but I missed the lifestyle and our house on the mountainside in the valley town. And as typical pattern goes, moms with a soft heart cave to their children's wishes, and we went back because of me. She thought with her heart, not with her head. Her child was able to override her higher logic with emotion instead. My older sister, my senior by a few years, knew better and she insisted she didn't want to go. My younger sister was still an infant and thus couldn't communicate her indifference or preference.

I carried that guilt for a while in my later teen years when Mom mentioned the issues we faced with Dad, and that it was because of me they had come back to the West Coast. I was the one who had insisted to go back.

Chapter 7

Predatory Cousins

1991

The year we spent on the prairies was the darkest time in my life, and what happened then would have repercussions on me for the rest of my life. For a few months, we took a trip to India—my mom's brother and I first flew overseas then Mom followed later. I had taken months of homework with me, which I completed, and was ahead of the rest of the class when I got back. They hadn't kept up with the cadence the teacher had assigned my work to me according to the projected progress anticipated.

During the India trip, my mom arrived during the second month that we were there. This trip was eclipsed with scarring, earth-shattering events that haunted me for most of my life. How I wish Mom had been with me there from the beginning, perhaps the outcome would have been markedly different. I fell victim to incest within that first month during her absence. At the time it seemed like child's play, but later the shame, guilt, and self-blame that the victim of incest feels eats away at them. The incest fact erupted violently six years afterward, during my first episode in senior year when I was committed to the psychiatric ward. I had finally told my mom years after it had happened. Older predatory cousins had found a great opportunity during this trip to India, during the initial time without my mother there that first month.

The incest perpetrator was an almost adult male cousin. This boy's older sister found out about the indecent play time and blamed me saying, "You better keep quiet." This mark will stay with you the rest of your life she had said. It was fondling, and for decades afterward felt to me as bad as rape.

This is a critical lesson for parents everywhere: Do not easily consider sending your kids alone on trips to visit extended family when they are young or even early teens, and please don't fully trust every relative. Statistically, the majority of child predators are not strangers but those in one's trusted circle. An empty mind is the devil's den for predators that see an opportunity and their mind goes south to perversion and fulfilling amusement – the convenience of it under their roof perhaps propels a whole set of twisted thoughts forward that never would have surfaced if the circumstances weren't perfectly in their favor. It could be a male or female perpetrator, a relative who is a cousin, an aunt, or an uncle. Is it truly necessary to send your child alone? Are sleepovers locally even necessary? The pediatric society of America says no; they specifically run ads on TV with respect to this topic saying these ventures aren't necessary.

The short-term convenience of sending your child somewhere, either for a break for yourself and/or for their enjoyment, could yield some long-term losses. Agreed, it's only a fractional percentage of time that this happens, but that percentage is there. It is a gamble, and the ideal conditions are present that create an environment to perpetuate perversion. Parents generally speaking are well meaning and protective of their offspring; they simply want their kids to have a fun vacation and send them with blessings and prayers. Never do they expect to get a child back who is secretly broken. Perhaps the continuous coaching during childhood of what is a bad touch versus a good touch is critical, and training the child and empowering the child to say a loud "No!" to the violator could be a deterrent as the violator may feel that the child is confident enough to tell the other adults of the invasion. I am thankful for the training schools give to children in grade school and I sincerely hope the awareness and such tips help deter this heinous crime of pedophilia. Tragically my parents with their limited understanding of school curriculum had opted out of the standard body safety standard training that was delivered to children in grade three at my school in the mining town. Had I been able to sit in that class it may have thwarted a bad outcome. I may have recognized bad touch.

My parents were oblivious to those pedophile risks; they trusted family completely. The thought of a sex crime never entered their wildest dreams, and even the expectation of full care was assumed by them, that there would be no neglect by an aunt or uncle. I haven't still ever mentioned to my mom a time of major neglect by another relative – I remember a time before this India trip, about four years prior, when I was about six years old: We had gone on a family trip to visit relatives in another prairie town. Our family never stayed at hotels; we always stayed with family as is typical in brown culture. Rarely do brown families stay in hotels when visiting other family. During this trip and after the week our family stayed when it was time to depart I decided I'd stay the summer there after the parents came back. I had insisted to the point of embarrassment for my parents and the hosts during our departure in the driveway. I had begged to stay as I was having a great time with all the children who lived there. This aunt and uncle had said to my parents that it was absolutely fine for me and my sister to stay, and my parents, perhaps not reading between the lines of these hosts obliging out of politeness – allowed me to stay.

In most regards, the stay was uneventful, thank the Lord. Again I was at the tender age of six years old. Perhaps for that reason I was awfully neglected. My aunt never had checked on me if I had bathed, and I ate cereal most days for breakfast, lunch and dinner. This was the staple food eaten most of the time at her house. All of us children ate sugar, sugar, and more sugar. Fruit loops, I remember—we ate a lot of those. My aunt was pretty lazy with her own kids, too, with respect to this area of food preparation. She also napped excessively during the day I noticed. My mom wasn't like this aunt at all; my mom only took naps when she had a headache.

During that vacation, I walked around in the same clothes all day and slept in those same clothes for weeks. I walked around this unfamiliar city's neighborhood, and the older boys living in this neighborhood, random strangers to me, would make fun of me—my messy hair that still had a bow stuck in it and was never combed. They also made fun of the black-white and velvet-silk dress I wore for what seemed like eons and never got out of. I'm surprised I didn't have a cloud of flies following me everywhere. Also I wore the same white knit leggings and these were badly ripped from the knees. Before I went back home my aunt made sure I wore the other undamaged pair of leggings in my suitcase on that last day.

Perhaps it takes a special kind of relative to care enough about these things when your parents aren't there. Delilah was with me just the first week after our parents left, she started to dearly miss home and was flown back shortly after expressing the desire to see our parents again. I had decided to stay though. I was the brave kid, I felt and told myself. In hindsight I realized this trip was riddled with child neglect to a degree once my parents left. Four years later far worse would happen during the trip to India that was also without my Mom's presence; a trip eclipsed by sexual abuse.

The incest that happened when I was age ten I hid for almost what seemed like a lifetime. This incest event may have been the catalyst for my bipolar onset in my adolescent years. This event created insomnia later for me at times in the years before the discovery of my bipolar disorder. Only did I confide this to my mother at such time when I no longer remained coherent and stable. Otherwise while in my full senses I was always tight lipped and guarded about this tragedy.

Between age ten and sixteen, a steel door went down in my head on that incest; never would I tell a soul as the boy's sister had coerced me to never say anything. Of course, there was collateral damage in it for her younger brother. If word got out, it would be bad for him, and she had to make sure she would make every effort so that the truth could never come out.

It turned out to be a dark year on the prairies, a time eclipsed by this incident. This was darkness of a different sort compared to the darkness of my parents' turbulence. This darkness was entirely mine and a burden I could not share, the guilt tormented me. I was a young mind with no understanding of these events – I did not interpret this incest as an event I was a victim in, but rather I interpreted it as one I was an equal perpetrator in. I had no remorse for myself when I thought about these horrible events overseas. I felt I had instigated the incest somehow. I felt I was grotesquely bad and dirty and just as much at fault as the others in that incestuous mess.

I direly hated the school on the prairies too. I missed the west coast. Sadly the only real thing I missed specifically was the mining town's mountain house. Mom and us sisters had moved back to British Columbia in 1991 as Mom gave Dad one more chance but this time everything would be on her terms.

As I'd mentioned before my mom had some conditions related to moving back. Firstly, she demanded the mining town home to be signed over to her sole ownership so that she would have an asset in case she needed it for her children financially if she found she needed to part ways with him again – he reluctantly signed it over. Secondly, in addition to the mining town home ownership change she required the family to settle permanently in Vancouver shortly after returning to the West Coast. Thirdly, Mom required of Dad to accept that Aunt Jennifer and her family would co-share the living space with us in Vancouver for added protection and stability if Dad became violent again.

So we left the prairies and went back to wrap up the mining town home and head south to Vancouver permanently. I wish leaving the prairie town meant that I could leave behind this horrific incident of incest but it tormented and followed me for years.

For a few years thereafter our family went through a series of reconciliations and break ups between Mom and Dad. It was very awkward for us in the community, as everyone in our church knew what was going on. Word definitely made its way around fast. These years were a pendulum of separation and get-together, separation and get-together for Dad and Mom. It continued to be quite the show for the Indian community locally – the gossip train went by us and around us. Dad's tempers would erupt and he'd rapid cycle between mania and depression again – sometimes working and sometimes not. It was very difficult for him to hold down a job with the depression surfacing. Mom had to continue to try to pull him up and iron fist him finally. She was seldom encouraging and understanding at this point. She had tried so hard already for years but circumstances and age had hardened her by now.

By this time my maternal Grandpa Samuel, had been widowed for a decade already after his wife's death. Grandpa stayed with us for a year or so in the rental home and also rode the waves of separation and reconciliation as he supported his daughter through it. In Vancouver we rented a bigger house to accommodate all of us; Aunt Jennifer's family, Grandpa, and us five. It would keep my dad in check, having other males there. After all, what would three young girls and a five-foot-two-inch mother be able to do to defend themselves?

Near the end of our rental home time, Dad showed some stability where he was no longer as much manic as he was depressed, and hovering right under the rim of normal, just slightly depressed, a part on the bipolar curve that maybe easier to manage by the family compared to full mania or suicidal depression. Mom had become a homecare nurse like her sister Jennifer and it was a good steady income job. She had qualified for a mortgage on a new place of our own so we could move into our own space as we yearned for the privacy of a family again. Just us like in the mining town, only this time would be different. Dad was on medication now.

During the property acquisition Dad forced Mom into a fifty-fifty ownership of the new Vancouver house as he said it wouldn't feel like home unless he owned part of it. He was only to be a secondary guarantee cosigner but then threw a curve ball at her while at the property lawyer meeting and refused to cosign unless he was made fifty percent owner.

She had paid for the property lawyer's time and felt pressured to close the deal and caved to his demands under time constraints. We had moved into the house and Dad started becoming hyper and on the manic upswing. Suddenly he felt like the authoritarian again with his own house and without Samuel and Jennifer's policing presence. Mom finally changed the locks while Dad was out one day and called the police, she wasn't going to risk regressing into the lifestyle of beatings again. The independent year on the prairies had made her confident and stronger in her resolve not to ever allow the abuses to reoccur. Mom filed a restraining order again, but this time at the Supreme Court level, an order that would not expire.

Chapter 8

Discovering I Was Bipolar

1996

The faint bright side in our move away from the prairies to the bustling west coast port city was that we were finally able to participate in a school that was significantly diverse. There were a lot of other Asians in our high school; this made making friends possible. Racism was starting to gain exposure as a bad thing, and you didn't want to be labeled a racist, not even back then. In our suburban school, ten out of every thirty kids in each class were brown. Our classes were sizeable. There was an explosion of immigrants in the 90s to this port city and it meant a high enrollment in our suburban schools. Delilah and I finally felt like we belonged and school wasn't dreaded as much anymore; we didn't continue to resent not being white.

I was hoping for a full-ride scholarship earned in high school that would foot the college bill. I didn't want to lean on my mom to pay for college. She had worked two jobs in the beginning when she finally evicted Dad. In those early years after Dad was no longer living with us, Mom worked at a twenty-four-hour donut shop, then worked at another fast-food restaurant, and drove us to school and back. Mom did this draining and hectic schedule for years. She felt more comfortable at the donut shop, especially working the overnight shift, as cops sat there routinely. Dad was always out and about wandering the streets with a restraining order against him. She was in constant fear typically but the cops' presence helped. Mom realized Dad was watching her from afar at times beyond the restaurant windows.

Mom was low on sleep always, taking care of a toddler and both of us older sisters in high school. Years earlier, when her and Dad were still together; she had a home care nursing job at the time of buying the new house, and my dad was working back at the mine and they qualified, based on that higher income level, for a larger mortgage. But then layoffs came across the home care agency, and Mom had changed the locks on Dad so he couldn't get in after another catastrophic fight. She was stranded paying for a home mortgage and tethered to her jobs. She was working a full-time job and a part-time job to make ends meet. If you have assets like a home in Canada, you are not eligible for the easy welfare money.

She did this nightmarish schedule of what translated to one and a half full time jobs for years, and then the fast-food restaurant chain saw promise in her, and she worked there until she retired. Mom was a dedicated worker who dealt with politics, staying on the straight and narrow always. Things bothered her about work and politics; it kept her up at night. She didn't have a safety net, another spouse working; she had to keep going. Don't let anything get to you. Keep moving. She ignored the drama thrown her way and stayed the steady course.

Mom's health was bad, she never had any time to exercise, her blood pressure would skyrocket, and her cholesterol was off the charts. She had bouts of situational depression, as the divorce lawyers took so much and she was stressed from being alone and a single mom raising three daughters. The occasional phone call from a sibling brightened the day. She also entertained a lot off and on, and people certainly took advantage. When relatives didn't want to cook in the evening, they'd come to our house for a meal. Internally I think she craved the adult company. Meats were expensive in Vancouver. I would be frustrated because we'd buy generic everything for ourselves. Forget ever buying some branded potato chips. But for guests a special lavish menu was prepared. She had to keep the reputation up she felt. She had three girls to get married some day. She had to be the hospitable hostess always. Also perhaps this was her time to shine her culinary skills. But most importantly I understand it now as the need for adult company instead of always surrounded by child obligations.

As a fast-food manager she worked for many years and was offered the regional manager position multiple times over her tenure. But every time she refused it, as she didn't know computers and didn't know how to spell. She didn't want to set herself up to fail. So she continued at the store level, even though her repetitive strain injury in her elbows worsened as she would jump in and help with the deep fryer when things got busy and the lunch or dinner rush started.

The company valued her in that she was an easy-going manager who could train other new managers. She loved feeling needed. She didn't mind the after work calls. There was always one issue or another on a daily basis that she would need to troubleshoot; when someone couldn't show up for a shift and coverage had to be arranged or a pipe burst at the store and a contractor had to be dispatched. There were the late night or middle of the night calls when an alarm went off at the store. Sometimes she would be sent to the bad part of town where it was a dangerous area, two hours of traffic roundtrip, and expensive gas which was never built into the salary factor.

Often she would get the challenging stores that were fixer-uppers; the kind of stores that were failing operations—high payroll, high food costs, high supply wastage. They would terminate the current manager and send her there. She was dedicated and devoted. It was her livelihood; there was no getting complacent at this job. It was the main income source.

While living our teen years at the Vancouver house, we had renters, but the rent didn't help cover much of the mortgage payment. Sadly but not surprisingly the renters would take poor care of the place. Mold grew in the dank weather of Vancouver on those basement windowsills and was never cleaned timely. Carpets needed to be replaced every time a renter moved, and entire unit painting needed to be done as well. My mom would be saddened at the windowsills being eaten away when she scrubbed them in between tenant moves. That was permanent damage. One renter would put his cigarette on the sill and use it as an ashtray. A giant hole developed. This house was my mom's prized asset that she had put her blood, sweat, and tears into.

There were some crazies who rented too, who she had to evict. One older man was having trouble opening the shower faucet on his first evening in the suite. Mom wasn't home when he had knocked and asked for help. Delilah was the timid one, although three years my senior, so I went to help him and the problem was the shower faucet's on/off mechanism. He was inebriated from evening beer consumption and took his clothes off in front of me and got in the shower. I was appalled and scared. Delilah told Mom what had happened when she got home. Mom was mad at me. "Did you have to go help him? You could have gotten locked in and raped. You should have known better. You would have screamed, and no one could help you." Her words hurt but were coming from frustration, fear, and the what-if of the worst could have happened to her daughter. She went to the basement and told the guy to get his stuff and leave. He nodded quietly, and the next morning he was gone. He had given Emilia a decoration piece, the one that is magnetic and keeps swiveling, and we threw it in the trash can, my mom didn't even want to keep it in the pile for Salvation Army.

We still had a second home in the mining town that wasn't selling and there was still a mortgage on it as well. The tenants in the mining town were also a constant nuisance. Mom couldn't meter the utilities; one set of tenants was a large joint family who were awfully wasteful in terms of running up huge water and heating bills. It was flat rent and the utilities were built in to the rent amount, to our determent. It was difficult renting out a home in the mining town in general, so we couldn't increase the rate or be picky with renters and setting rules.

Mom would run up to the mining town, a day's drive from the mainland, to repaint the home when a renter left. She was amazingly efficient at rejuvenating the place every time. Mom could do the entire house with one bucket of paint. She said if she contracted out the job, it would cost not only fees but multiple buckets of paint as the painters would not be as careful with the usage. She'd do very thin coats with the utmost care and frugality.

Out of curiosity sometimes I look back at the mountainside house on Google Maps in that beautiful mining town situated in a valley between mountains and that is also adjacent to a large lake. This lake would freeze over and pickup trucks would drive over its ice to shortcut their way to the other side in the deep winter. There were steep, evergreen-covered mountains on both sides with the city in the middle, and some houses were built up the side of the mountain. We were lucky to be on Thirteenth Avenue.

When I looked at our old home on Google Maps' street view, for the first time after decades I almost fell out of my chair. I lived there? It looked so small, like one of those houses in the run down part of town, the simple four sided structure with minimum walls within. But it was in fact a small three-bedroom house with a giant triple window in its living room. It probably was less than 1,600 square feet, with a basement we would rent out to tenants which would further reduce our living space. But this was me in my thirties looking back at that home, now living in a 6,000-square-foot home with Darrell. As a child my old home seemed palatial. Your world as a child adapts quickly to all it knows. My dad had bought the home for $42,000. We sold it for $116,000 in the late 90s as a fire sale during the divorce settlements. The house next to us had sold for $139,000 before the mine shut down. My mom was devastated as the timing hurt us. We had to wait to sell it as Dad had put a lien on the property for many years, thus we had missed the opportunity to sell it at a bigger gain.

The divorce lawyer had taken thirty thousand dollars from my mom by the end of the five or so years of the legal battle. She didn't qualify for legal aid because of her house assets. My father's lawyers were two young Indian men, who were good at what they did. They were garnering sympathy for him in court from the judge very effectively. "Look at him, Your Honor, in those dark glasses. He is broken, ill, and depressed."

My mom had asked a friend for a lawyer referral; she didn't even know where to start looking. She had just minded kids and worked at a restaurant most all her life. Looking at the *Yellow Pages* frustrated her; it was overwhelming. Mom's friend got her husband's business lawyer to gladly take the case. It wasn't his area of practice, but this lawyer saw money. He could barely keep up with the family lawyers in that courtroom. He could not get his words out in time or be aggressive enough as the family lawyers who were well trained in this area of law. It wasn't the business lawyer's lane to be taking such a case anyways, the right thing to do would have been for him to refer the case to another lawyer in the area of law specific to Mom's case. After the case ended, the old lawyer took a trip to the French Riviera and died there from a heart attack.

The legal battle over property settlements went on for years. The 1990s was a time of calls from the payphones of downtown Vancouver for my dad. Often the calls would go to the Vancouver home's landline where us three girls and Mom still lived. Dad still considered himself married to Mom and didn't care that the local courts had served him divorce papers; the divorce wasn't on church paperwork where the original marriage certificate had been put into place overseas long before so the local order was invalid to him in his mind. The church only had the power to void this relationship, not these local, pencil-pushing courts of the state, he felt. Delilah refused to ever see Dad; she was attached and devoted to Mom. She'd seen and felt her pain vividly those years in the mining town.

Despite everything, my mom always told us girls, "He is your father. I cannot change that, and I never will. You see him if you would like to." Emilia and I would see Dad. He'd take us shopping but never give us cash; he feared we'd give it to our mother. We really only went for the shopping. His lectures were long, but the gifts were enticing. I was going to milk his money as much as possible, as he never paid child support. He wasn't going to help Mom in the least; he was suing her over property. He'd put a lien on both the Vancouver home and mining town home. Mom couldn't even sell the homes and go on welfare as there were those liens in place. She was tied to working and weathering bouts of depression as the seasons came and went, and loneliness for companionship persisted.

My Dad eventually opened up a convenience store, as he always wanted to be a businessman. He dreamed of it and becoming a millionaire. He was hit as a pedestrian in a car accident and received a thirty-thousand-dollar settlement from the lawsuit. I'm not sure if it was a frivolous case.

With the funds Dad had bought a failing convenience store. He chatted too much with each customer, and lines were long. He'd get previous day donuts from restaurants to sell with hot coffee in the morning. He'd sometimes sit in shorts in the walk-in freezer at the back of the store since it was hot and not air conditioned.

One time I visited him there, and a lady said, "Are you his daughter?"

I said, "Yes."

She said, "He's really nice, and he needs you guys, he misses you."

He lost the store; he couldn't manage it. He was taking medicines subsidized by the government so there was that stability factor but he was likely sleep deprived making those early morning donut runs. I am not sure his health status at the time of the loss of the store. But I'm sure customers started avoiding the store. It wasn't a good convenience store anymore if it wasn't convenient to get in and out of.

These years were filled with anxieties. There was a sporadic presence of Dad only when us girls obliged the stressful interaction. Then the final straw of anxiety was grade twelve, when that full-ride scholarship to be earned in senior year never happened. The scholarship applications never got written. But my episode did happen. And it shattered my straight A running; my perfect grades were gone and transcripts tarnished.

School was a successful time before the final year of high school – I had friends and also academic success from grade eight to grade eleven. But then grade twelve, which was the final most important year, started – and so did the slow onset of my very first bipolar episode. I was sixteen. I kept sinking steadily into depression prior to entering the hospital that December. In the fall it was a slow ramp-up, or perhaps ramp-down I should say. I had stopped eating, stopped sleeping, and words weren't processing anymore. I'd stare into space.

It was a steady decline into this slow motion state, triggered by particular events I speculate. There was a continuum of failures that led up to the hospitalization.

I had excelled in school in grades eight to eleven. My mom was one who was not happy with a 97 percent grade; where is the other 3 percent she'd ask? Mom never helped with homework, she didn't know how to and we never asked for her help either, we knew she wouldn't know the answers to any of the Math, English, Science or Social Studies questions. I think kids have it in them to set their mind to books and learn on their own at home if they are utilizing the school resources during the day, outside of those with learning disabilities where significant assistance is needed. I was the first and only one to go to college on my mom's and dad's side, out of the cousins, besides Uncle Christopher. My mom told me while we lived in that crowded basement on the prairies when I was ten, "Alayna, now do good in school. You could have a great job like Uncle Christopher has in Europe." He was an accountant and traveled and had a great lifestyle with abundant money.

Uncle Christopher was attached to Mom who was close in age with him, and as the decades passed she became modernized in her thinking, relatively speaking, compared to her other brothers and sisters. Most of Mom's other siblings were too traditional to go to a modern wedding where there were Indian women in strapless clothing and drinking alcohol. I loved my mom for attending Uncle Christopher's girls' weddings later in the 2000s. Mom was open-minded enough by then, not prude and all too traditional like the other siblings. She was the only one of six other siblings who attended his children's weddings. Uncle Christopher came in for Delilah's and my weddings, which were a week apart. Mom wasn't going to miss his kids' weddings either. Uncle Christopher and Mom often talked on the phone, keeping in touch. He, after all, had been her confidante over the phone in those early years of marriage when she didn't tell her parents what was going on, but she had told him everything, as he was the only other sibling who was also abroad and removed geographically from the rest of the family.

I was intrigued by Uncle Christopher, the only sibling of the eight who had left India and gone to college. He had taken the chartered accounting exam but not passed. Aunt Jennifer told me that little talked about fact later. But he still had a great job at a publicly traded company. I was encouraged to strive as hard as he did, and so school was full of good grades including the critical subject of math. Later in life I thank Mom for having me strive harder and not accepting C's and B's in school from me, as it made me not go for a simple job but a license I could fall back on.

I had many successful years of high school behind me but the summer break before senior year the reality of bipolar disorder hit. It started its slow climb, a time when my mom took my older sister to India to get her married. Delilah had liked a white boy from school, and that wasn't acceptable to Mom; an Indian boy would only do. It was unacceptable to marry outside the ethnicity; you'd be disowned and bring shame to the family. The overriding sentiment was you would also sabotage your sisters' possibilities from being considered for arranged marriage. Thus mom forced Delilah away to quickly get an arranged marriage to a man overseas recommended by Aunt Jennifer's then husband.

My mom's brother from the prairies came to stay with Emilia and me during that summer. While Mom was away making wedding preparations with Delilah, I was difficult with our Uncle.

I was already working part-time and grown up enough I felt; plus on some level I loathed men. I was taking care of my younger sister, Emilia, who ended up going to my aunt's for a couple weeks after my mom departed to India with Delilah.

The summer before my diagnosis, I had gotten myself into a hit-and-run accident, and I was the one who had run. I had a loaner rental car, as my mom's car was in the shop. I hit my school counselor's car while making an all too hasty left turn. I turned the car and sped off in the opposite direction. The counselor had followed. I gave up after twenty blocks and some turns, finally stopping; he was tailing me successfully. I got out and apologized. I was profusely embarrassed.

There was a student in his car, a former friend of mine from the previous group I had left who I had been awfully mean to. She watched, and I was feeling so exposed. To me she had been a needy one; I resented her weakness. Her brother had committed suicide years prior, and she wanted everyone's attention I had felt. At least that was my juvenile mind's belief about her. As I grew older, I realized how naive and ignorant I once was as a high school student with too much judgmental starchiness – and I feel I grew more compassion for other's circumstances only later in life.

The counselor let me go without exchanging insurance information. He said, "It's fine. It's just a scratch, but don't ever leave the scene of an accident again in your life." I was shaken because I had a rental car that was already fairly bruised and dented, but I didn't know whether I could hide the dent from the shop when I turned it back in. The day I had to return the vehicle I had an on-call shift as well at the retail clothing store I worked at. In retail that's when you don't have an official shift, but you call an hour ahead and ask them if they need you and show up if they do, based on foot traffic of customers. I had never had one on-call shift materialize into an actual shift in my two years there, but ironically this time I was called, and I hesitantly told the manager I just couldn't attend the shift. She was irate. I learned later in life I had trouble recognizing authority, as I didn't have a father, a typical trait that sometimes runs with people without a father figure in childhood. I should have been more respectful of the boss's need at the store for help.

I told the manager about the accident and that I had to return a car to the shop, and I had called so many other colleagues to take the on-call shift for me earlier, but it was a beautiful, sunny summer day. No one wanted to take my shift. I knew I had to return this rental vehicle without it being detected that I dinged it. That's all I could think of in my slightly episodic mind – I was utterly fixated and obsessive about the car's damage. I could not resolve myself that it would be okay to wait till the next day which was a Monday (the shop was closed on Sunday) to turn the car in and still attend my shift. I had prepared myself to take the car in that day and have an excuse memorized that the dent was already there if the car shop had said anything. I was a nervous wreck. I had rehearsed the potential conversation over and over again all night in my head. I couldn't have a work shift throw me off my memorized plan.

The decline to come in for the shift was the turning point for the retail manager. Refusing the on-call shift the day of the shift meant disciplinary action. The next regular shift I went into I was informed I was fired. It had been a prestigious retail job at a company that was selling high end designer brand clothing; one where I was the envy of all my peers. My head just wasn't in the game though. It was difficult for me to lose my retail job, it had become a big part of my identity and the reason I was in a popular group at school as of the last year or so. Failure was difficult for me; there was a lot of fixating and obsessing over such things. The retail manager was looking for an excuse already to be able to fire me. My productivity had declined as my mind became unfocused that summer, and leading up to it I had gained the animosity of my coworkers.

I had no idea initially on why the animosity existed. My colleagues hated me. A vicious rumor flew that I had reported the sexual orientation of one of the associates to the locals, and they had threatened him because it was so taboo in the 90s. Gay and then Indian gay was absolutely intolerable to the conservative minority, which was fast becoming populous and the majority in Vancouver. They had projected into the future that within a couple decades, whites would be the minority in Vancouver. It was a giant immigrant hub and port city. The 90s was dangerous for the white LGBT community; for Indian LGBT it had to be tenfold worse.

I had told a mixed brown-white friend at school that my coworker Rocky was gay. She had had a crush on him previously when they attended a different school together years ago. This was too much information for her to handle, so she leaked the information further to her thug posy, and the threats started against Rocky. I had leaked a secret to make a friend closer to me, because that was what high school girls do; they confide in one another, and that makes a better friend. It was an egregious error.

This instance had translated in a twisted and morphed manner back to the clothing company in that I had directly pushed people to threaten Rocky, as he started to be harassed for being gay by multiple Indians locally. At the time retail stores had gay men working there, but they definitely had to be secretive. Even cosmopolitan Vancouver in the 1990s had incidents of gay men raped in alleys. My colleagues hated me, and they made work very difficult for me. I never figured out why, until I had a conversation with one person who I started with—there's always a special bond with the person you share a first day with. I approached her and had mustered up the courage to ask her why there was so much animosity, and she uncovered it for me. "Alayna, you told people to beat up Rocky for being gay."

I deeply regretted sharing anything about Rocky's orientation to that mixed girl who I was trying to deepen my friendship with. The news had been exaggerated horribly as it came back loudly that Alayna wanted Rocky beat up. Rocky was the brother I never had—humorous, outgoing, loving, nonviolent—and I really loved him as a coworker and person. He treated me with respect. Gay men make great best friends with their additional dimension of perspectives. I regretted telling this mixed chic his situation, and it was later interpreted as though I had directly facilitated the angst against him from the community.

Years later I ran into Rocky at another retail location of the clothing company. I gave him a hug, and he was shocked and laughed it off a bit at the public awkwardness of it. He was my Secret Santa the year before I had been terminated. I gave him a card with an apology note embedded in the holiday card, and a tear streamed down his face when he read it. Sitting there at the party, it was a silent exchange between him and me. He was a lovely soul. How I wish to see him again, ask him how he is doing. I hope he was extremely successful in life and found his happiness and soul mate.

Rocky had transferred to a new location while I was still working at the company, away from the conservative suburbs. I continued to be loathed by the staff. My gestures of goodwill to him never got communicated, but he didn't need to communicate it to the rest of the staff. I had made an error, and I suffered the resentment, unfriendliness, and ostracization from coworkers for another year before termination.

I was direly confused every time I worked a shift; it was fast becoming a hostile environment. I thought at first it was because I wasn't a size two, like most of the other girls, or because my skin was breaking out badly. The other retail workers made a point of letting me know how much they hated me but indirectly so. The managers also hated me as they learned I was allegedly a gay basher. When I refused that on-call shift, it was the opportune timing to get rid of me. I'd worked there two years, ancient and tenured for someone in retail.

I'm glad I did pester the manager for a reference letter afterward, attesting to exceptional and solid sales performance, as this was a place where I'd excelled at selling eight-hundred-dollar leather jackets and I had done phenomenally sales quota-wise. That reference letter helped in later job searches. At this high end clothing chain the regional heads had valued my sales record and dispatched me to other stores to work outside just my home store. It certainly felt more like home in those other stores, as the staff didn't treat me in the same marginalizing manner. But if coworkers in the other stores thought I was a gay basher, it would have been just the same frigid coldness as experienced in the home store. Sadly this retail job, which started out being a cherished and wonderful place for camaraderie, quickly turned into an environment where I dreaded each shift. The animosity of coworkers waited for me every day I worked and their remarks and bullying continually grew in frequency and ferocity as the months went by – until the finality of my termination from the company.

 I was terminated in August, and went into a steady depressive decline over the fall where a comatose state took over. By December my mom was beside herself speculating I had taken drugs and perhaps that was what had rendered me incoherent and lethargic.

 I had also failed my first driving test with a dangerous move in an intersection. I had learned driving street style, no lessons. Delilah had taken lessons; I was saving my mom's money by not buying lessons and partly I was overconfident that I didn't need lessons. I had profusely complained to my mom for weeks when that failure had happened and she was irate that I hadn't gotten over it quick enough. She was perplexed at how long lasting my fixation over the failure was.

 These were the events of the summer of 1996. I had failed the driving test, lost my job, and gained my mother's disappointment over handling things poorly while she was gone to India. It was a horrid summer indeed. I didn't realize that my circadian rhythm was starting to dial away from me and my brain chemistry was starting to become imbalanced. Neither did anyone around me imagine that I was having this mental decline that paralleled my father's. After all I was a straight A kid. I was an honor roll student, every year. I found I had attained one of the three highest grade percentage positions in the class in the instance the teachers would disclose rank to the rest of the class. Teachers back then would do this to foster a sense of competition in the students. I was highly competitive; my mom had made me that way. Losing the job and failing the driving test was too much for me.

In the fall I had regressed as the final year of school started, and my mom came back from India. By winter I was in the hospital. Mom was resentful of her siblings. "You made my daughter crazy!" she told them. In her mind she knew the summer without her had been a rough one, and her initial reaction had been that it was my fault, but later when I started my mental digression she realized it may have been external factors contributing to the decline, such as treatment by the rest of her family that was to take care of Emilia and me.

Upon her arrival back, my uncle had complained to her about me, specifically that I had told him not to put a wet towel on the door but to hang it up to dry elsewhere. I knew from past experience that my mom would rip into us kids for doing that—the moisture ruins the wood by expanding it. So I asked him if I could hang it elsewhere for him. He made it a thing later to tell her I was rude about telling him to remove it. Then the fact I wore a robe after getting out of the shower was apparently inappropriate to him. I was shocked and confused that he brought that up to my mom and their other sister. It was a full length robe. Later in life I figured it made him uncomfortable seeing me in a robe.

My mom's oldest sister also chimed in with her issues. I never liked this sister of hers. Emilia had gone to live with this aunt that summer after the first couple of weeks. I was frustrated and saddened to see her go, but it was a good thing she went. She was only fed ramen noodles by me at our place. I was just a kid myself. But she resented cleaning her aunt's toilets. She was only nine, and we never made her do that task at our house. These were the things we never tell our parents until older age. My mom would have been livid had she known that Emilia was made to clean the toilets at her sister's house, who had six almost adult children of her own and were well capable of handling this task.

Later my mom felt my aunt and uncle had created my mental instability but not before admonishing me for their complaints originally upon arriving back from India. I was still functional in early fall and so it was interpreted as my fault. The bipolar diagnosis was yet to be made later that winter. Here was a third compounding failure I felt, that my mom was utterly disappointed in me upon arriving back from India. I was made to feel I had created a hot mess of family relations and acted inappropriately while she was away.

I fixated on those losses; of Mom's disappointment with respect to strained family relationship, of a job loss and of driver's license failure. I told my friends at school I got there too late for the driving test, and I had not ended up getting tested. They laughed. They had asked, "Did you fail?" My face went beet red and they saw right through my lie. How it irked me to ever fail. The bipolar mind fixates on things to an incredible degree. Failure becomes an obsessive point.

I had handled the household with my elementary school sister in tow part of the time, during the summer of 1996. When school started and my erratic behavior was reported to the principal, he took me aside and asked about home. I said, "My mom can't make it here to the office. She's in India." He learned I was home alone with my sister. I never mentioned my uncle; I hated him. Uncle had gone to stay with his oldest sister anyways after the first few weeks.

The high school principal was in shock, kids alone with their mom on the other side of the world? But he didn't call child services. I was driving by then. I was an honor roll student for years now. Also I was a thoughtful artist with beautiful real life drawings and sculptures that still adorned the art classroom even years after creation. I had taken responsibility quite early to run outside errands and get my little sister to church on Sundays. My mom needed us to be self-sufficient, scratch having an adult with you while you drive on a learner's permit even over four lane narrow sharp turn high speed bridges. I had also been working a part-time job for two years at an upscale clothing store in the local mall by then. The principal took a calculated risk and let the matter go that I was on my own with my little sister who was by now back at home with me so that she could walk to her school every morning alongside me. I'd demonstrated sustained academic success and he might have had some remorse at the level of responsibility I'd assumed. My mom was to be back soon anyways.

    The chronology of failures on my part finally reached an inflexion point where the downslide was uncovered one December night during the time Emilia had a friend come by for a sleep over. I had awoke in the middle of the night and said, "Mom, the cops are outside. I can hear their sirens." This was the same night that while Emilia and her friend were horse-playing, I said, "Don't play like that with each other," as something in my mind blipped over the incest.

    This young white girl who was still in elementary school immediately realized my fear and had somehow the wisdom no one in my family had honed in on before. She pointedly asked me, "Did something happen to you when you were young?"

    That is when the memories slid forward like an avalanche. I was shocked and dumbfounded. This little girl had just hit the nail on the head and let the genie out of the bottle that was trapped for years. My incest history seemed right out there hovering above us all at that moment. That same night I went into Mom's room, and she realized I was hearing things that weren't there, like sirens that I said I heard but no one else did. I was traumatized and numbed by the secret that this stranger in our house had uncovered in a moment and that later escaped my lips. I had told my mom about the incest the very next morning.

    That Saturday morning after Emilia's friend left the memories of the sexual abuse violently erupted into pressured speech while my mom sat across from me. It came out in a jumbled and somewhat incoherent manner. My mom didn't seem to understand at first. Maybe there was some underlying shock that she was trying to absorb. She had some cognition of what I was trying to tell her I'm guessing now. I remember sitting in Delilah's bedroom when it all came tumbling out. Delilah wasn't there, she was still overseas and newly married, but unhappy.

I recall vividly back to that snowy day, my mom didn't know how to react to the news of incest on that Saturday morning. She hit me, saying, "You are pregnant, aren't you? You slut!" By Monday I was in the ER. She broke down in tears that Saturday morning, knowing in her mind it was true—the incest—and cried. Her gut reaction initially was to deflect it.

She had started to take what she thought was remedial action immediately. She'd ragingly ripped the pictures of all our male cousins in front of me, and it should have ended there she felt. That was to be my therapy. The inferno of rage and injustice should have subsided with those pictures that went into the trash. But chemistry in the brain doesn't allow sleepless depression's train to halt after just a conversation or such actions of some pictures ripped into pieces. I was to get over it and certainly stay quiet on the subject. This whole situation would bring shame, and I'd never get married. She didn't realize I needed therapy.

The mind's vault had opened during my episode. My mom tried to teach me how to cook on Sunday and left for a church meeting. In hindsight I'm sure she needed to regroup inside her head and thus left for a few hours even after learning of this catastrophe that befell me. I looked at the stove and didn't know what to do with any of the ingredients. By Monday morning she realized I wasn't coming back into my own; and she didn't have me go to school but took me to my family doctor, a lady physician whose clinic was open that early Monday morning. The doctor had told her to take me to the emergency room immediately after her and mom talked a while looking over at me and I wasn't very responsive to the doctor's questions. I was staring into space and utterly detached. Maybe it was drugs, my doctor seemed to say to my mom. Maybe in the 90s the doctor had already started to see depression cases in children more frequently. I don't know what her and my mom discussed other than instructions to take me to the Emergency Room (ER) immediately.

The ER had tested me for drugs. They quickly realized after the test came back negative that it was acute depression and a psychiatric matter. There is a pediatric wing at hospitals and my mom asked the doctors to put me there. The staff had said no. Maybe there was no room, or maybe I was too old to be in there with the younger kids. It wouldn't be safe for the other kids perhaps they thought. So I went to the non-lockdown side of the psychiatric ward where adults stayed. Memories were made there that haunted me for decades.

There I was admitted to the hospital, the scariest experience as they don't have a pediatric section at the psychiatric ward. I was in there with men and women. The bedrooms are gender segregated from one side of the wing to the other.

There were four hospital beds to every room. One night a man had walked into my shared room. He was struggling with his own monsters. The nurses pulled him back to the men's wing. There was a geriatric age woman in my room who, in the frigid winter months, would keep the window open. I could barely sleep a wink even sedated because of the cold. I would toss and turn in anguish. I think she was suffering from hot flashes in hindsight. But I didn't understand this then; I was frustrated and upset. So at one point as she slept I timidly closed the window next to her, and she instantly awoke and ripped into me. I reopened the window immediately for her. It was a nightmarish experience full of restless sleep.

There was an Australian lady in the ward who I remember vividly. She had a scary laugh and crazy-eyed look when she stared at me. The look where you see the whites all around the pupil, eyes that are all too widely open. I was both in awe at her confidence and scared of her too.

There was a gentle old lady there as well, in pink silk robes. She reminded me of Rose on *The Golden Girls*. I called her Grandma, and she would mention me to her family over the phone. "Such a sweet African girl." I was amused at that. Maybe she needed glasses and didn't have them with her or had lost them.

My mom was saddened to put me in the hospital, but what could she do? I was hallucinating, seeing things that weren't there, and had debilitating depression. Even in depression there can be symptoms of psychosis. This was the only episode of the six I'd had in my life so far that started with sleepless depression and not mania.

The incest from age ten was a major catalyst causing the slow mental breakdown I speculate but I can't be sure that was the sole cause. I had weathered many years with that gruesome knowledge inside, and if I had the self-awareness of it having a lasting impact in my life, after the December hospital admission I may have talked to a therapist about it on an ongoing basis. But after two meetings with the counselor that early spring season, I figured I could move on.

During my time in the hospital my sister Delilah came back hastily from India. Delilah had been overseas and newly married, and I missed her greatly. Maybe that was part of the trigger of the first episode, not having Delilah around as a support. Delilah came back after my hospital stay, and I was elated. She was like Mom. She felt even more like Mom, being married now and a woman in my eyes, not just an older sister. She was only nineteen at the time. History had repeated itself; my mom married at nineteen and my sister at nineteen as well. This marriage would last only another six months.

Delilah was married to her first husband less than a year and ended it after arriving back to Vancouver with him. The cultural barriers were too much; he was too odd. He smelled, his hair wasn't right, but in my head he was a nice guy, but I wasn't living her life. Perhaps it could have worked between them but I'm not sure as someone looking in from the outside. She hid him from her friends. She didn't take him to parties. Earlier I kept telling Delilah before she went to India, "Don't say yes to this. Stick up for yourself if you don't want this!"

Delilah felt guilty; Mom had done so much for her girls all her life and asked Delilah to comply with the arranged marriage. Mom wanted her to forget the white boy she loved dearly. Mom pressured her and guilt tripped her. I remember Mom stroking Delilah's long straight hair, saying, "This is my good daughter. She always does what I say." One time Delilah's tears streamed down silently. Mom pretended not to notice and walked away.

An older cousin had pressured Delilah to approve of the arranged marriage as well. They were friends, she told my sister: "Look, if the door is open and you don't go out of it, that's a worthy feat. If the door is already forced shut, it's no feat on your end to resist the temptation to go out." The outside was the white boy in our cousin's figurative analogy.

In mid-January after a three week hospital stay and Delilah helping assess and support me daily I went back to high school – but in an embarrassed way. My friends came to visit in the hospital; everyone knew. In honors English class, they all clapped when the teacher welcomed me back. I felt I was judged however. Maybe it was sympathy in their eyes and heartfelt kudos that I had survived a challenge, not snide judgment. But at the time their temporary attention to my plight gave me an inferiority complex. Years later I found out there was another boy and girl in my graduating class, whom both ended up on leave from school for mental illness. Bipolar incidence is one percent in the population. My graduation class was about 250 students. That roughly corroborates the same statistics confirmed in studies.

I think about these other two children and me, and how the statistic seems accurate. I read somewhere that one in every one hundred is a psychopath in the general population. But is that Venn diagram mutually inclusive between those with bipolar disorder and those labeled as psychopaths? Psychopath is such a poorly coined term. It is an improper one, used to label someone's personality dimension negatively. I have medicines that read they are in the antipsychotic class of drugs. Unfortunately every time I read about this class of drugs I have to push out of my mind the 'psycho' morpheme. The main distinction between bipolar disorder and any other mental illnesses is the psychotic tendencies of mania. Thus *antipsychotic*, as coined by the medical community and pharmacies, is the medicine used to counteract mania. Hopefully the medical community will eventually come out with a new term for these medicines because the psychotic term may never dissipate from pop culture and always will be associated with serial killers in news and media.

    Winter of 1996 started with many weeks in the hospital, after which I dusted myself off. By January of 1997 I was back to school in my grade twelve year. I was in what the counselor called 'audit' status with various courses as the teachers let me sit in and see which courses I wanted to do course work for and finish for a grade, so there was no unnecessary academic pressure put on my mind to take a final exam and finish a course. I still finished a handful of courses albeit with lower grades but was elated to get into a university, not just a community college. However I couldn't continue the straight A running needed let alone shoulder the original elected course load which had consisted of Biology, Chemistry, Physics, and Honors Math that would have helped qualify me for a scholarship. That ship had sailed on me completely.

    I sat in for auto shop class during that spring semester of grade twelve as it seemed to be an easy course to handle. I also still wanted to be the son that Mom never had and change the oil in her car and use a jack. But when I stood on the lug wrench to unscrew the bolts in the tire, the boys all laughed at me. I must not have been more than 109 pounds, as I'd lost weight during the long depression. I tried to get the lug wrench twisted by using my arm strength but finally I tried by standing with both feet on the wrench. I was a laughingstock; maybe the boys were just genuinely amused in a good natured way. I was embarrassed and felt I'd made a fool of myself and that their laughter was sinister.

I also once had corrected the auto shop teacher when he had spelt "jewelry" wrong on a slide. It was an overhead projector slide about belongings not to be left in a car. The boys laughed then, too, and the teacher just smiled. Next the boys had yelled in an artificially high pitched female voice, "Mr. Miller, it's *jewelry* with one L, not two!" That was it for me. I dropped the class shortly thereafter.

I also audited Grade Eleven Psychology, but the teacher took me aside and said I knew too much for the good of the other students. He told me to read the *Devereux Scales of Mental Disorders (DSMD)*. "That's your level." They were talking about light topics in class like moods while you are driving down a scenic road and fluffy discussions like that. I was pulled from that class. The other kids thought I was pretty cool, a twelfth grader in eleventh grade psychology. The teacher was the school counselor who I had rear-ended the summer before. I sure hated him for pulling me from that class. I figured he was intimidated because I could teach it better than him. After all, my mind was not fully recovered in terms of judgment after the episode. I felt I was the subject matter expert on psychology. If only they would let me skip to the psychology twelve course. There, the kids would feel safer with me and I could contribute in a more valuable way with my own experiences of mental illness, and at the same time do so without disclosing to those that still didn't know that I myself had been suffering from what they were learning in their textbooks.

Once I graduated from high school, I held a series of retail jobs within a span of a few months. I was still trying to find my focus, and I worked at a sports retail store in the summer and took grade twelve physics in summer school. It was said to be the most challenging course in all of high school; I barely passed. I'd smoke cigarette butts that were on the ground at recess, using my own lighter taken from the kitchen junk drawer to relight these smashed butts. That's probably where I picked up a cold sore, which erupted decades later.

I had picked up smoking at age fifteen from a cousin who taught me and another cousin how to take a long inhale and feel the buzz. Unfortunately, that high was enough to hook me till age twenty-four. In the years to come, I'd buy single cigarettes off of people in college, as buying a pack made me feel so guilty I'd want to finish it immediately via chain-smoking or give it away, which I did so many times. I prayed earnestly for God to give me the power to kick the habit.

The series of retail jobs I barely held in this post-episode year were a stark contrast to my first job ever when I was in grade ten. That particular job was in professional services. A couple years before senior year in grade ten we did a job shadow type internship and were allowed to volunteer shadow (unpaid) for a couple weeks in an industry we chose. Most of the people in my class picked retail stores they were vying to work at some day. I figured I wanted to be a lawyer, so I asked for a law firm, and I got placed at one. That helped get my resume to the top of the pile as related to a multitude of retail jobs later over the years. Such part-time jobs I typically would jump from and resign, but I got fired from a fair share of them as well.

The law firm was a good experience but it was a shock to them when they found out I was only in grade ten. The firm had thought I was in college. The office manager skimmed over my file. It was free help! But when I started there they thought I was a very slow girl, as I didn't know anything about office supplies, filing, answering a multi-line phone, or transferring calls. This all changed as a week into the job when they discovered my true age. I had interjected I was born the same year that the partner had just stated he graduated college in; everyone stood still in the mail room and were shocked during this conversation. They were all exchanging glances with one another as their jaws dropped to the floor. Suddenly they didn't let me walk alone up Granville Street in the dark and they would take turns dropping me off at the SkyTrain. It was a complete switch in attitudes, where there was disappointment before now there was gratitude at my skills, for a tenth grade student, I was poised, professional, and killing it. They got me the best-ever butter wafer cake for a going-away happy hour—nonalcoholic happy hour for me of course—in their conference room. I couldn't find the likes of that cake ever again. Also we'd play *Doom* on the computers after hours, me and two other young lawyers. It was a happy moment in childhood, and I was set up for success, as showing law firm experience would instantly get you into any retail place that only saw non-professional experience with other applicants.

This early law firm job I had done so well at was a stark contrast to the retail jobs I tried holding down years later after my episode in the summer following graduation. These jobs were a complete failure as my commission earning abilities were not there anymore, neither had good judgment and focus returned completely even a half year after being out of the hospital. The medications were still a moving target to get the right doses and types for me. I would doodle on pages near the retail store's cash register while I was supposed to be greeting customers that were trafficking in routinely. My mind would wander endlessly and become easily unfocused and distracted. During that summer I barely focused through the summer physics course too that was just in the mornings.

Once winter came things felt better and more stable however – I think my brain and the medicines had found their equilibrium point and optimal balance. I enrolled for the January semester of college and was looking ahead to the beautiful college campus on the mountain top. I had a successful first year of college at this local university halfway to downtown Vancouver.

To save bus fare, I'd hitchhike from the place I parked at the bottom of the mountain, on the street that wound its way to the school at the top. I wanted to save the bus money for when I might need it to buy single cigarettes from people on campus but they seldom ended up taking my money and I'd come back home with most of what I left with. My mom was beside herself when I told her about the hitchhiking. I had to tell her as she questioned why I still had the bus fare money when she checked in if I needed money from her purse. She told me, "I'll give you the money; I always do. Just don't hitchhike." But that was Mom's hard-earned money. I always had some guilt. Especially since I was buying smokes at times. I needed to save what she gave me for what I really needed and find other ways to save, so bus fare seemed discretionary to me. I worked in a daycare on the college campus for two hours a week eventually, which earned me sixteen dollars each week, thirty-two dollars biweekly. It was awesome; life was starting to feel good. I was studying, experiencing college, and able to have a coffee and smoke in privacy on the mountaintop.

In those college years, I used to carry my dad's pocket knife he left behind. Having this made me feel safer while traveling home in the late evenings on the SkyTrain. The ironic part was the blade was so tight, I didn't know if I could get it out quickly enough if I needed it in an emergency. Delilah had been mooned on the SkyTrain once by a drunken guy. She never took the train in the evening again. She had bought a used car instead as she worked full time at an electronics store and could afford the purchase. She had vowed never to travel public transit again. I had a plethora of night classes, and it was a long day sometimes too. Mom's car was used by her more than full time job entirely so was unavailable to me. So public transit was the only option and I figured I could handle it, Delilah had always been a lightweight for challenges in my mind. One semester I managed to get all my classes into Tuesday and Thursday only. These were long days. Travelling back in the dark with the sun down, that knife made me feel invincible.

I was into a third semester straight, I had taken three semesters consecutively without breaks since starting and a full course load of five classes. Each course was three credit hours, so I was earning 15 credits each semester whereas most of my counterparts took only 12 credits. I had the dream of finishing early before four years as I had already lost some time and started half a year late after finishing high school. I begged Dr. Singh to take me off my medicines; it didn't appear I needed them anymore. I was studying and working at the same time and seemed one hundred percent normal and successful at what I did. Dr. Singh was not a psychiatrist but a primary care physician who my dad saw. I wanted a female psychiatrist initially, but when they couldn't refer me to one and we just couldn't find one in the *Yellow Pages*, I settled for Dad's doctor, an older man who was also originally from the subcontinent with a mild demeanor and very caring mannerism. He'd do a lot of research on the side to brush up on psychiatric medications.

Before I started to be in the care of Dr. Singh I did briefly see another male psychiatrist, Dr. Patel, who was my care provider right after my first episode. I only had two appointments with Dr. Patel and discontinued quickly with him. It was uncomfortable as a female victim of incest; talking to a male doctor. I asked Dr. Patel in the second meeting, "Can you refer me to a female?"

Dr. Patel jovially replied, "I'll change my sex!" He had smiled and closed his door, ready to prep for the next patient. That was a frustrating response to receive; he didn't address the issue at all or help refer to another provider.

With Dr. Singh, though, his short height, older age, and mannerisms seemed mild, easy, and nonthreatening. He was not intimidating in the least – both in appearance or personality. There was something about him. He was fatherly somehow, and I convinced him to take me off the medicines and that I was fine now. So he said that maybe this was a onetime episode, perhaps just depression, and consulted with my mom, and she wanted to believe it was temporary too. If they saw depression again they would put me on medicines. I'm not sure the rhyme or reason but I just wanted to not take medication anymore and be completely independent of them and have back what I thought was a true sense of normalcy. Taking the pills once daily was upsetting. Even when everything seemed fine; it just didn't make sense to me to continue to take them. So we hastily stopped the medicines. This was yet another naive mistake my mom and I jointly made. Perhaps she had gone with emotion again instead of logic. She knew how much it meant to her child to be off medication, and part of her may have wanted to believe it wasn't a permanent condition like bipolar disorder but just a one-time mental breakdown.

Chapter 9

Psychiatric Lockdown Ward

1998

In our overly optimistic thinking, my mom and I settled that my first episode was just a bout of situational depression and nothing permanent. But very soon, I was to learn I had bipolar disorder for life and that it was a very permanent condition.

Initially I joined university thinking I would do every summer semester and finish in two and a half years. I had already lost the first half of a year upon graduating high school as we waited for my summer school results to be in and I felt I needed to get caught up with missed time. My mom had worked so hard. I wanted to be that son for her, and become a Chartered Accountant in Canada, to make it possible for her to travel, experience and enjoy life to the fullest. I wanted my mom to not have to work in fast food anymore but live a glamorous worry free lifestyle. The timer was on, and I needed to get a job and earn. I was focused and determined. But then winter came, and I started the skin medicine Accutane. It clears acne but at a high price; skeletal hyperostosis is a risk, blindness is a risk, and you must abort any pregnancy that happens—you sign that before taking the medicine. Otherwise the child will be severely deformed when born if you take this while pregnant. In the late 1990s, they didn't know this skin medicine also interfered with the delicate psychiatric balance some have. In later years it was discovered that children had committed suicide and been plagued with depression because of the drug; at which point the drug company quickly corrected the marketing of the drug to only those not struggling with mental illness or those without history of mental illness in the family.

    I had started college in spring of 1998 and by winter of 1998 after three solid college semesters I was full-blown manic. My mom heavy heartedly called the doctor with news of my instability as I didn't want to go into his office. I was put back on medicines, some were new this time. But one gave me such dry mouth, and another medicine was a generic brand version this time as opposed to the original I had taken a year earlier and it gave me a horrendous after taste that would be nauseating for hours. I refused to take this generic one but couldn't articulate the reason why as I was fairly unfocused and jumping from subject to subject rapidly, which only made matters worse. My mom was desperate to get me back to normal; she even sent me to my uncle's house on the prairies as a break from school as she figured that would help and that perhaps it was partly the school burn-out and stress feeding into my mental regression. But I was psychotic with my uncle and only friendly to his white wife. She was relatable in my eyes; she understood me I felt. But she also had no skin in the game, she wasn't as worried for me as uncle or mom were. My mom had to fly in and take me back. Years later I was ashamed; I'd wasted her flight ticket money while I looked back at this episode in disgust of myself. She hadn't planned to come out there but had to buy an expensive return ticket last minute to bring me back. I was compounding the expenses on her unnecessarily.

    By December I was going to parties, drinking, and dressing promiscuously. With bipolar disorder you take risks when episodic, but God saved me every time from true harm. I had just enough sense not to get into an irreversible decision. My mom and dad came together at this time on my situation and tricked me into going to the hospital. They had lied that a close family friend was very sick and admitted to the hospital and that we had to go visit immediately.

    Once you're in the ER, you're locked, as I was an involuntary committal. I remember the nurse had scolded my parents for lying to me. I was angry at them for years, but now realize they had done the right thing; I would not have gone voluntarily until it was far too late.

Drinking as an Indian woman was strongly frowned upon culturally, and I reeked of alcohol when I entered the ER. My mom's oldest sister had arrived in the ER waiting room, to be a support for Mom. I gave my aunt a hug and suddenly she held her breath and made some immediate judgments. Her son had been forward with me; he wanted to marry me someday, something I laughed off years before—gross, he's a cousin, we don't do that, not me certainly. I'm sure he'd disclosed this to his mom at some point, as I reported to my mom he had called me from the gas station he worked at one day and told me so. Well, this aunt was immediately judgmental; I could see the invisible thought bubble above her head—where had this girl been all night?

She figured her son would be overly desperate to ever show interest in me again.

Earlier that day I was trying to get home via the usual bus and SkyTrain route. I had lost my bearings and ended up finding the help of two older men working in the trailer office at a junkyard in downtown Vancouver. The junkyard was near the water, and you could see the mountains in the distance beyond the strait. I remember the frigid temperature, the sun blinding my face, and those immovable ice capped mountains that witnessed so much.

The men let me in from the frigid temperatures; I begged them to. They were reluctant and apprehensive at first, as they knew it would look terrible to have me sit there with them. But finally they realized I'd freeze out there and it would become a bigger problem. One customer walked up, a burly man, and said, "What's going on in there?" I'm sure it looked awfully sketchy. Customers seeing a young girl through the glass, sitting at the desk behind these men, in party clothing and a coat to partly cover it. The customer must have thought they'd hired what looked like an under-aged hooker.

The party the night before was in an art studio in the warehouse filled industrial district of Vancouver, just up the street from where I sat now. I left there in the morning. The lady who owned the studio arrived that morning and was distraught when seeing the damage created there on the walls by the partygoers. I remember in the middle of the night the bathroom seemed grotesquely dirty to me and I was throwing hot water on the walls and floor to dissipate the urine from places. The studio owner's wall paintings were sideways, but I couldn't recall any permanent damage to the place. My mind was racing. I remember the music bringing tears to my eyes the night before, uncontrollable crying. People at the party were watching as the DJ continued his beats; I could feel their eyes on me. Also I was unnecessarily protective of a young high school girl ready to leave with an older boy. I'd asked him with a sharp look, "You'll take her straight back to her house, right?" Foolishly putting my business where it didn't belong.

    The sun was up in the morning when I tried to find the bus stop but couldn't. The alcohol had worn off; I hadn't had too much. It was frigidly cold but the sun was bright and blinding. At my low weight, even one drink was enough to inebriate me, and Mom never had alcohol in the house. I never built up any sort of tolerance to it. I was a lightweight for drunkenness. But the episode going on in my head was in full swing, and I couldn't think straight and talked extremely fast with the classic pressured speech of mania. The junkyard men let me into the trailer which I was thankful for, and I was able to call my mom. Mom told me in a calm voice that my dad was on the way. I was scared when she said that, why was dad going to arrive instead of her? Would he be irate and angry and try to hit me? But when he arrived he looked sad and defeated. He only spoke in a calm voice and looked at the ground most of the time.

    I didn't realize mom and dad had been in touch as of the past few weeks again because of my illness being uncontrollable now by mom alone. This was a turning point for Dad too. He had always been in denial of his own illness, and now his daughter exhibited the same erratic behavior he was told he exhibited but never had believed anyone. A stone wall of realization had hit him. This illness exists. It is very real. How can I ignore I have this when my child suffers from it as well? I've passed this on. I need to own this now, and get her out of this before it's too late for her. I need to put my differences aside with Lydia now and just focus on my child surviving life and coaching her. These may have been Dad's thoughts.

So my Dad drove down to get me, he didn't have a car. I noticed as the driver got back into the car and drove away that it was a fellow student from my university he had driven down with. My Dad had gotten this student's number somehow and scared this boy who looked like a jackal with his tail tucked between his legs. The boy quickly dropped him off and drove away. This was the boy who, the night before with his sister, had gone to the party with me. They had left me there, as I was a loud manic, and it was embarrassing I'm sure for them, I speculated. This boy was going into actuarial sciences, a Jewish boy who lived in the British properties, the most expensive part of town. Him and his sister thought I must be very weird or drunk to behave that way, and they weren't having any part of it. Or maybe they had told me they were ready to leave and I had waved them off. I never asked my mom how they ended up dispatching this boy. I'm speculating Mom must have retrieved the number desperately from outgoing call display on our landline phone and gave it to my dad to call this other student. No doubt my dad likely threatened him into taking him to the closest junkyard where he had dropped me off the night before.

I know I had acted bizarrely and said things that were completely on tangents while at the party. The embarrassment and deep regrets stay with you for years until you forgive yourself. It's not you; it's the illness. It's not a character flaw, it's a brain ailment. It takes a lifetime to sometimes realize that. But some never accept this and never forgive themselves. They take it to the grave that they were somehow faulty, broken, and worthless.

I spent three weeks recuperating in the hospital. On my birthday, I had been admitted to the hospital. My sister Delilah had thrown me a party at home and had made many dishes. She knew I was going through a hard time but wanted the affection to show through and bring me back into my own. The invites were out, but only one friend showed up, and this friend was confused where everyone was. Only Delilah and Emilia were home with the lights off. Mom was at the hospital with Dad and me. All the other friends stayed away, as they realized I was episodic. They were a fake group of friends. A group of 'friends' I had jumped into quickly and always was hoping for their acceptance but not fully receiving it. I had wanted to be in their popular group so badly. In grade eleven I had left the misfit group behind when I had a fight with one of the overweight girls in that group who always complained about her weight. When I finally suggested lifestyle changes, her world bottomed out, and I became the vilified person she complained about to everyone. But despite this lash out, I realized in later years, the overweight friend was a much truer friend than this new superficial, surface-level posh group. She was the only one to come visit me in the hospital this second time, and give me a stuffed toy I still have kept to this day.

 I had invited this snooty popular group of girls to my birthday during my second episode and they never showed up. They knew I was in a manic phase. These cliquey girls were close-knit, and I was the tagalong only during those last couple high school years. They'd talk fast, back and forth in Korean, and I'd wonder if they were talking about me. One time I mustered up the courage and asked, and they looked at each other and said, "No, it's about this weird boy in the halls."

 This so called 'weird' boy had come out of the closet years later, and the high school boys at a reunion said, "Gross, what if he was checking us out in the locker room?" He was a good kid, and he wanted to be in a boy band. The New Kids on the Block and Backstreet Boys were a huge thing back then. Everyone dreamed of going stateside and making it big.

This cliquey group of girls was all honor roll recipients and ran the student council – one of them was the president of student council in fact. They were smart kids who wore nice clothes and seemed classy. I worked at the high-end fashion shop in the mall during the year I joined their group, maybe that's why they let me join – I worked at a designer brand store. But I was always struggling to keep up. Never fully secure in my relationship with them. Always wondering, always trying to perceive if I belong. That was the last year of high school. I kept in touch with some of them. And they all bailed on my birthday. Except there was one Middle Eastern friend who showed up, but she wasn't in that popular group. Not even a call to me from the others to say, "Sorry, we won't make it." Or that "We feel you need help." I had talked to their ringleader a week earlier and was going a mile a minute. She was the informant most likely to the others to deter everyone else from showing up. Better they didn't show up anyways, and better yet I wasn't at a party honoring my already grandiose mind and making a fool out of myself. Delilah told me about my middle eastern friend coming by and being the only one to knock. It was a sad realization; don't ever try to belong in a group based on their popularity and outward appearance. If I'd invited my previous group who I saw as misfits they would have certainly come to my house, and the overweight friend who heard through the pipe I was ill and in the hospital visited me and we regained our friendship. I had not invited her to my party since our fall out years prior.

    So my birthday came and went with only one friend knocking on the door at home while I was in the hospital emergency room and being involuntarily admitted as a psychiatric inpatient. The ER nurse had given me an injection for sleep and it sedated me for 14 hours. I had hid a lighter in the Emergency Room in my brazier and the ER nurse was shocked to not catch it until I had to change into hospital robes. She was disappointed in herself, shaking her head and told me she could have lost her job for missing that. I'd handed it over to her hours later in the ER room myself while changing into the hospital gown before sedation.

In October the onset had happened with Accutane in the mix, and by December I was sleeping little to none weekly. I think in a week I slept maybe five hours total across the seven days.

This time the psychiatric ward experience was not so shocking, even though it was a lockdown where you couldn't leave the wing without a nurse escort. I ran the show in the ward amongst the other inpatients. I was still all too grandiose, as I was coming down from my episode. I was vibrant and articulate, but I was a manic spectrum individual amongst mostly depressed individuals. The people who I met there I remember vividly even to this day; their unique personalities and how life had brought them there. Since I was an involuntary committal I could not leave on my own accord. A committal like this means someone else had brought me there and I hadn't walked in myself. That's why I was in the lockdown ward and could not leave the wing. Later, they upgraded me to the non-lockdown psychiatric ward when I started to show more stability of mood.

In the non-lockdown psychiatric ward, folks are gentler and not so deranged. In the lockdown ward are the harder cases—suicidal or harmful—where they are shaking off the worst of their ordeal in that area first.

I was in there with a man who had cut his arm off below the elbow. He was a bald, young biker. His arm was operated on and sutured, but then the second step was admittance to the psychiatric ward. This man was depressed and would cry silently in the corner. His other arm was covered in tattoos. He would smoke heavily when the nurse would take us out. We all would look forward to the smoke pit outside, even in December weather. This young man's dad was just as broken as my mother. My mom and his dad would exchange some words of understanding. My mom felt I'd cut something of myself off too; Alayna was sick a second time, and that meant she had it for life. She's cut out that robust future we thought she'd have. Mom's world had bottomed out from under her this time; clearly this illness was forever.

    I sat in someone else's bowel movements during that stay; some are still struggling and not fully medicated enough to regain balance and cognition. I guessed it was the lady with schizophrenia who laughed uncontrollably and asked me if I'd killed someone. I had sat on a stretcher that was by the elevator as we waited to go downstairs, when my fellow inpatient said, "Wait. Stop. What is that? Careful!" I fell ill for a couple days after that incident, although I had quickly gone to hand-wash my pants and showered. Maybe the feces had contaminated me somehow. I hope it was just a seasonal cold. Those memories were disturbing. But later the people stay with you and their life stories linger in your mind. Their wide-eyed looks where you can see the whites all around their pupil, that same crazy-eyed look I remember seeing there two years prior. If I reflect now it reminds me of a druggy with their pupils dilated and eyes open too wide while walking into a convenience store in the wrong part of town. In some situations it might just be a full-blown manic sufferer.

    I came out of the hospital rebalanced and sleeping right, but then the slight depression that comes after a manic episode started to hit. It takes three to four months to find my bearings each time. Back to full normal takes time, although you feel normal soon after the sedation and mania comes down. But to acquire the same level of judgment as before the episode and drop the giddiness, only time brings that back. Especially if it's had a ramp-up period and sleeplessness of that long. In my later years, I nipped it in the bud faster as I had five sleep medicines on hand, along with a meticulous self-awareness that grew over the years. Later in life I anticipated when I had to increase my antipsychotic medications at certain turns in life for a few months and then go back down to the baseline dose when things normalized. Especially around the mothering years of sleep deprived nights.

At that Vancouver hospital, my mom's world was shattered. She could only take a few days off at a time. There was no *Family Medical Leave Act* (FMLA) equivalent in Canada back then or disability to care for a loved one; such allowances legislatively came in later years. The company didn't offer disability unless you directly got sick. My mom's many hopes for me to complete my degree, have a good arranged marriage, have a successful well rounded life—were gone. Mom was broken over it. Only the last resort and traditional remedy remained, and that is if a girl won't finish school, then get her married. Culturally this is the next logical next step. We didn't have enough money to pursue a Mrs. Degree for show and a better suitor proposal. A trip started to be arranged by Mom to take me overseas until I was engaged there and could come back only after being betrothed.

There were no other options in Mom's mind. Alayna couldn't have a cousin marry her, although some were previously interested. Now she had a tarnished reputation.

I would have never gone for a cousin, but now I was guilty and desperate. I was this growing liability on her hands. She sent me to India for ten months, until I was engaged. I was nineteen. My fiancé was older and partially bald. I broke off my engagement in my third year at the university, after being engaged about a year.

I was doing a bachelor's of business administration with accounting major and then on track to write the four-day Chartered Accountant exam. I was in the midst of starting an internship and then post graduation I had planned for an auditor job to acquire my years required to earn the license of a Chartered Accountant.

In the third year of college, my confidence came back. I was in my youth, fit, and healthy with a waist that stayed at twenty-five inches and an hourglass figure. I was insulted if they didn't turn and look, which they always did. Even women couldn't help but look, and the convincing part was when women couldn't hold their stare to your eyes; they had to sneak a look down. That was a compliment when women did that.

I was accepted to one of the largest Multinational accounting firms with offices worldwide. I felt more sure about myself than ever before. These factors cumulatively brought the confidence in me to break off my engagement over email with my fiancé in India. He had only been some sort of band-aid fix to a problem my mom was trying to solve.

My first fiancé was itching to finalize marriage paperwork after I had left India, so that I could legally sponsor him. He was shocked when I broke it off. He had emailed me once, telling me he thought about me all the time and it was driving him nuts. He had consulted an elder on this tormenting matter, and the man said he needed to reduce contact with me, so it would help alleviate the issue some.

I am not sure why I said yes to the proposal while in India, maybe it was because I was still immature and marriage seemed exciting. But from a pragmatic view he was also the only option amongst various more conservative suitors that had come forward. My mom really desired me to be engaged before I came back to Canada and this was my ticket out of there.

I was staying with my mom's youngest sister the majority of time while in India. This sister had a joint-family system, five families all in one giant concrete mansion. During my ten month stay in that Bombay mansion, there was a middle aged man living there as well with his family. This middle aged man was a complete drunkard who limped because of a car accident injury years prior and had a wandering eye. He was married with three young children. He had been a creepy, perverted uncle type and been a bit too fresh with me, putting the moves on me over that summer, and I rejected him pretty plainly with a slap in front of his wife.

I had a great amount of satisfaction in slapping this man across the face in front of his wife. This occurred when I told his wife he'd been inappropriately forward with me, and she had looked at him sharply with an inquiring but not surprised gaze.

She knew he was sleazy. I remember vividly we were on those stone baluster railing terraces they have in India, this one was facing the east, and the bright morning sun hit us all, but it wasn't sweltering hot yet. He said, "Alayna is a liar." That's when he got my right hand coming into his left cheek as he faced me. I wish I had throat punched; but I hadn't thought of that instinctively like the slap. Slaps seem too temporary a punishment in retrospect, a punch would have had some lasting pain.

He was a horrible person who gave his wonderful, faithful wife a lot of angst. His wife was elated and so was her family – at the fact that I'd slapped him hard. They knew this man had a wandering eye and was flirty. Of course his immediate and extended blood relatives were embarrassed over the situation. They couldn't meet my gaze for weeks. I left India a few months after that, once I was engaged. I left with pride reflecting on how I had handled that particular pervert in life.

This twisted man had found an opportunity to retaliate by putting something in my fiancé's ear after I had ended my engagement to him. My X-fiancé had commiserated broken heartedly to this man (whom he was loosely related to) after my breakup with him. They sat together not too far away from my former fiancé's house in the outskirts near a brick-making yard. This man had told my X-fiancé that I was interested in him instead, and that's why I broke it off. It was a completely false and certainly grandiose accusation. I'm not into the limping, drunk all-day, unemployed, father of three, already married type.

So I was briefly engaged to an overseas balding man and broke off the engagement a year after returning from India. Being engaged was the only way my mom would have sent a ticket to me in order for me to come back from India. I recall I kept begging my mom at intervals throughout the months during phone calls (that were only made weeks apart given international call rates) that I wanted to come back. I thought to myself, I'm sick of living with your sister and her boatload of kids. I never told my mom that though; she wouldn't have it. Saying something rude about her sister who graciously had hosted me for so long would be insolent.

India had its mixed bag of memories for me. Some good times, some bad times. I had my first pet in India. It was an English Pointer puppy who was just a few weeks old. One of my uncle's dogs there had had a litter of pups and I brought one of the female pups with me from his house in Delhi to my aunt's mansion in Bombay—it was a long commute. I fed Tesla like nothing else. I had named her after the Latin alphabetic character. Tesla dined on milk, meats, and all the luxuries most animals didn't get there. She was probably in the top ranking as one of the most fed dogs in that third world country, I could bet.

But my aunt was sick of the feces on the terrace. I wouldn't let Tesla go down to be with the other larger dogs that barked menacingly at her. These were large German shepherds. My aunt declared two weeks in, "Alayna! Your dog has fleas." She sent the servant to get flea medicine, and my dog was taken to the back of the servant quarters.

Tesla yelped for an hour strong and then her barking became weaker – completely subsiding shortly thereafter. Everyone had said it was just burning a bit, Alayna there is no need to go down. I fought with them; I needed to see her! I found her dead an hour later. There are antiquated ideologies in those countries that dogs are disposable similar to domestic animals such as chickens, goats, etc. I cried over Tesla's death. My aunt was chuckling alongside her sister-in-law, her reaction confused me greatly; she didn't understand my love and value for the dog's life. I had asked the matriarch of the house, my aunt's mother-in-law, where I could bury Tesla. In the meantime, my aunt had already had the puppy thrown on the cart of the refuse collector outside the gates. I asked the servant where the bottle was. He showed me, and it was rat poison.

To this day I have regrets. I should not have insisted to keep the puppy but sent it back to Delhi where Tesla's mom and siblings were, to my uncle's home that welcomed dogs. Fur babies have low value and are disposable to most of the masses in the subcontinent. However the upper-crust, modernized people there are different, placing heavy value on pets' lives, similar to North American philosophies.

The incident of Tesla's death and its regret crept up on me unexpectedly again when I was in my mid-twenties, and another bout of crying on Tesla's plight took over me. I had a total breakdown that my husband had to shake me out of, over the memory of her. It just randomly came on while I was cleaning the dresser mirror. My daughter was then only a toddler and I was in a new city, new apartment, and had started a new job at that time. It was an emotional outburst but a cleansing of sorts. It had just then dawned on me ten years later that my aunt had poisoned the dog. She had not mistakenly ordered something she thought would work for fleas, the rat poison order had been intentional. I was too young and not street-smart enough to understand at the time it happened, perhaps trying to see the good in people always. Naivety in young people has its own beauty, its innocence, but it is easily exploited.

In my forties now, I can clearly feel with sounder judgment that this was 100 percent on my aunt. Not on me. I had guilty regrets for many years. I should have sent the dog back. I should have stayed with the dog and trusted my instinct, and when I heard her yelping pushed people aside and went down to her. I should have been at her side when the so-called flea medicine was put on her and washed it off at the first sign of discomfort. Everyone that kept telling me the dog is okay were in on the mean prank to eliminate her and the waste on the terrace that annoyed them even though it was picked up quickly and the stone washed afterwards.

Since then my aunt has had a roller-coaster life with her seven children. Her kids had marriage breakups, with abusive spouses dotting their history, most never could finish school, had drug problems, etc. I have difficulty feeling empathy for her after her cold hearted action towards an innocent life.

I still remember Tesla. She'd sneak in through the loose wooden doors bolted together at the top and sleep on my pillow. I'd wake up to her low purring.

India was a ten month visit that was full of memories that would stay with me for a lifetime. I am glad I shed the baggage of the marital engagement when I came back and regained my confidence. After resuming college I realized I had regained my abilities and landed an internship that would help continue the path of Chartered Accounting. The excitement and glamour of the initial engagement ceremony had worn off and the more I integrated back in Canadian mainstream society my first fiancé had seemed antiquated and backward. It was becoming a situation similar to my sister Delilah's first husband from overseas, whom she had hidden away from the world when he got here as she could not relate to him.

Mom was upset at my engagement breakup but she was hopeful good things awaited and that I would land a great job and perhaps an even better soul mate in life. She had secretly hoped for one particular family in the US to ask for my hand in marriage, a family whose matriarch was Bethany and someone Mom would talk with off and on throughout the years – they were very distantly related generations up, not close enough to call it a cousin relationship. For years now she would talk with Bethany and she noticed Bethany specifically would inquire about me every time in relation to my plans and how my studies were coming along. She hadn't popped the question but my mom always had a feeling. Mom remained hopeful perhaps I'd finish college and be successful and maybe one day Bethany would ask for my hand in marriage for one of her sons.

I started interviewing with accounting firms during third year college after enrolling in the university's internship program. I had been a late entrance to the program, I had no idea the program existed previously. There were no mentors around in family or friends that could have told me about the internship sooner. I don't recall seeing it in a pamphlet but just word of mouth through other accounting students in third year led me to realize this is a great resource to help land a permanent job and I immediately went into the coordinators office for more information on interning.

My mom was new to the corporate scene and all she ever had seen of it was on TV and that which was overly dramatized. This had shown through in her misplaced concern during my interview process; I remember I was invited to an evening social event by one of the large accounting firms that were interviewing me. They had called all their potential candidates to a restaurant bar/pool hall. My mom was so nervous. Mom was tormented by the recollections of seeing on TV all the reported assaults on women in the corporate subcontinent, and also what they dramatize in the fictitious Bollywood movies with corporate India as the backdrop. She felt the interview might be a bogus ploy at kidnapping. She told me to decline the evening event, and warned me that this could be a fraudulent setup, where you show up to a false interview and get assaulted behind closed doors. But I laughed it off. "No, Mom, it's not India." At that time her concern was annoying, but now her concern I am touched by. I understand as a mom for your daughter you'd be scared, although her concern I felt at the time was misplaced geographically. She had said okay to the evening event but made me promise that I would turn around and leave immediately if it seemed like a set up.

Years later I recalled her fear. When working on the East Coast, I had heard a woman was assaulted by a stranger in a skyscraper building in the Washington, DC, area in her office while working late, by then it was the 2000s. It was shocking, a violent crime in corporate America in an office setting. Perhaps Mom's concerns were not that left field anymore.

I had landed an internship at one of the largest multinational accounting firms after the interview process. I think I was on the B list though, perhaps others had declined the offer and then they had moved down the list to me. I was a team player but I was book smart, not street smart. I had difficulty interpreting the grey areas in audit, where things aren't so black and white. I also could never read between the lines. At least while working in corporate Canada my mental health was never off kilter. It was a great time working in a professional space again after the brief work at the law firm I'd worked at in grade ten. This time I was an adult and felt independent and finally back in my own completely. I had been able to unburden from the incest secret and still be a proud member of our clan as I was the only one other than Uncle Christopher who had finished college and been able to land a white collar job.

Chapter 10

Arranged Marriage

2002

My husband, Darrell, and I aren't related. Not really. Grandfather Samuel's half sister, Bethany, would call Mom on occasion and specifically ask about me. How is she? How's her schooling going? Bethany's family was impressed that none of Samuel's grandkids had gone to college except Alayna. The reality was all the working age grandsons were cabbies or working at a gas station or trucking, and all the working age granddaughters were housewives.

Bethany had a boy who was four years older than me. This boy I fondly remember when I went to Delhi at age ten and saw him for the first time. I was an ugly duckling, but he was the kind of guy who would push weights, eye-catching, and attractive. He eventually went into the School of Engineering. My cousin, who at the time hadn't immigrated to Canada, was with me. She joked with me while we lay awake co-sharing a room, as we had to spend a night at his house while commuting between cities. She had whispered jovially, "So you like him? Hmm. You think he's cute, right?"

Thirteen years later we were married. Darrell and I were engaged for eight months. Bethany called and asked Mom for my hand in marriage. No down-on-one-knee proposing in our culture, at least not in those days. It would have been surreal if Darrell had done that for me but perhaps unnecessary I also realize. I call it "semi-arranged" because we had seen each other briefly that summer and were able to talk as family friends. He liked me, so he told his mom, Bethany: "This is the one."

At the time of receiving the proposal Mom had requested a few of her confidantes to pray for guidance on whether it was a good match, a customary thing done in the culture—look for a sign. One of Mom's sister-in-laws had said, "Lydia, I had a dream that our dad was sitting on the hand-woven bed in our village back home, and he was talking to someone else out of vision's site and said, 'This will be a good match; this should be done.'" Grandfather Samuel had died of blood cancer years earlier, when I was around twelve years old. He had become a heavy chain smoker in the last few years before he died. I'm glad for that dream my aunt had and for the message he left her. I don't think I could have ever written my life's account without Darrell's support and stability he provided over the years.

My grandma Edna died in January, a few short months before Darrell and I were married. Edna always thought it was my mother's fault how my dad ended up. When she died was the second and only other time my dad had hit me as he flew into a rage when I defended my mom from his verbal insults at the funeral. I was the brave sister so I couldn't let myself or my Mom down; I would get in the middle of them. I always had when I was there witnessing physical violence between Mom and Dad.

Delilah and I would have been the only grandchildren Edna would have seen get married. She would have seen my sister's and my weddings back to back, as they were one week apart, both on a Monday because rates were cheaper at banquet halls on Mondays.

There was one exception with Edna not having the opportunity to see any prior grandkids get married. She refused to go to her male grandchild's wedding that preceded Delilah's and my weddings the year before. He was also one of the eldest of the cousins, his mother, Dad's oldest sister, had married and had kids early. This cousin of ours was going to marry a non-

Indian outside the church community. You were excommunicated from the church if you did that as a woman; for men they had to convert their mate to the church's system and were allowed to marry outside with that condition. But this super progressive Middle Eastern-origin girl wasn't going to convert. Both my dad's brothers tried convincing our cousin to not marry the girl. They tried persuading him, explaining to him the marriage wouldn't last even five years.

The girl had a strapless dress on for the wedding day. We weren't invited because my mom was divorced to my dad already, but I really wanted to see her. I'm sure she was very cool. Grandma Edna would have been horrified had she went to the wedding, the bride in an off-the-shoulder dress? She'd shudder and make the sign of the cross; that's the devil there, that type of dress.

Our cousin is divorced now, twice divorced. His first marriage didn't last more than six months. But Emilia, Delilah, and I always speculated he was a hidden, untreated person with bipolar. He was awfully erratic and moody and couldn't hold down a job, just like me. His second marriage was to another one of his first cousins on the same bipolar paternal side of ours. Bipolar bloodlines crossing again can heighten the danger of increased probability. They did have children, and I say a prayer for those children that all stays well for them genetically.

I always had mixed feelings for Grandma Edna. She had her favorites; she treated us differently—my sisters, my mom, and I. We were not of her favorites. Edna had said in the hospital, when Emilia was born, as she held her, "Gosh, would it have been horrible if God had just finally given us a son?" Mom was enraged, sitting on the bed, exhausted after a C-section. She was seething with anger and never forgot those words about her daughter and Edna expressing disappointment while holding Mom's infant.

Since Mom had divorced, Dad would go to his mom Edna's residence often, who lived with her other two sons, rotating back and forth between their homes. It's typical for Indian parents to live with their kids. It's reconciled as your parents took care of you the first twenty years when you couldn't fend for yourself, so in their last twenty years they need that help and security back.

Both of Edna's daughter-in-laws, whom she lived with, would often retell the fact to my mom for years after Edna's death, that Edna often regretted not being good to Lydia, especially in Edna's final years. Edna had misunderstood. When she finally saw firsthand one of my dad's violent outbursts toward a son-in-law, where he was to maintain a level of formality, then it clicked for her. There was something truly wrong with him. Men hit their wives all the time—she, herself, was beaten—but this man was talking to his sister's husband, full-out yelling and wanting to swing at him.

They say Grandma died with that regret. She should have understood my mom's situation better. Dad was next-level unstable. If Grandma was more supportive, I would have remembered her fondly, but all I remember is her favoritism toward my other cousins who lived there in the lower mainland. Edna would look at me and my sister Delilah and sinisterly point at our long skirts and high-tops and tell her other granddaughter how we looked inappropriate and promiscuous. "Don't you do that, dress the way they have."

I don't remember much about Grandma Edna other than the negative; it's sad, really. She was the last grandparent who was alive for decades after the rest of our grandparents had died. It should have been a cherished relationship. She was the Grandma who was there in the same city with you, which is typically a blessing but I never got to experience her in a positive way even though she was always within reach.

Grandpa would also hit Grandma Edna a lot. The village watched I learned. It had become learned behavior on my dad's part; it was an acceptable norm. Grandpa's new wife Edna was thirty years younger, and Grandpa had a temper. His first wife had died when he was 45. Edna thought hitting was acceptable. But when Dad was aggressive toward another male, especially a sister-in-law's husband you typically don't have clout with, as relationally there is a handicap, being of the girl's family's side, that was when Grandma realized her oldest son truly had some sort of mental issue. She would have otherwise treated us with empathy for the decade prior to her death, but she lacked the understanding until that incident.

Grandma became free of grandpa's rage when he died in the 1970s. They said he had his mood swings, but above all it was noted as an immense anger. He was born in 1910 and murdered in the 1970s. Grandma made it to January 2003 and Delilah's and my weddings were just a few short months thereafter but devoid of all grandparents by then. Delilah and I were too afraid to allow Dad at our wedding. We thought he may react to someone or other or fight with relatives as he was notoriously known for and we would have been so embarrassed in front of our new in-laws. In hindsight there is a level of non-erasable shame and regret in our decision to not invite Dad. But we had made a decision based on those circumstances at that time, and using historical behavioral patterns as an indicator of what should be done. So our dad continued to wander the downtown streets of Vancouver as we celebrated our weddings with family and friends. Uncle Zachary gave us away, dad's brother. He was always there for us, fixing our furnace and other urgent matters as they came up over the years. He felt a strong sense of reasonability in that if his brother wasn't able to take care of his family that he would step in for emergencies. He was a support for Mom as a confidante to assess how Dad is doing and what current conditions were like.

Darrell was the best thing that ever happened to me. I prayed for myself while growing up that I'd find myself a better life, and a great life partner. I hoped for an equal in education and career caliber. I didn't want a cab driver, like many of the local girls had to marry out of their existing proposals, or a man I had to sponsor from overseas. The sentiment with us first generation Indian girls growing up in Canada was this: It is better to marry a factory worker from North America than a doctor from India. The girls I knew strongly felt this in every fiber of their being and I was the same way – there was definitely a strong preference to marry an Indian boy who was already settled in North America and relatable culturally. It complicated matters that it had to be an Indian boy as the pool in North America was limited, plus compound that with he had to be of the same religion.

My Dad told me I had hit the lotto with finding a spouse. He thought because of my illness I'd never receive a suitable proposal, only a cousin as an option. In fact Dad had pressured Mom to have her ask her oldest sister for her son's hand in marriage after my second episode; he was desperately trying to find insurance for his daughter's future. Traditionally it is a rarity for the girl's side to propose instead of the boy's side. It is also sadly seen to be an act of desperation. Hopefully society progresses forward to drop the notion that when the woman or woman's side of the family initiates the proposal it's a sign of devaluation.

My sisters were so excited for me. Delilah was divorced, and there had been no suitable proposal for her yet, and until she was married, I wouldn't be able to marry as she was older and my mom was worried if I married first she would become a spinster. One of my cousins on our maternal side, for years, had been trying to get Delilah on board for marrying her husband's brother she would need to sponsor from overseas. Delilah wasn't having that again; the last one that was sponsored ended badly. She felt the cultural barrier was too much and so she had rejected that proposal for years. But now there weren't any other options.

Darrell and I would talk on the landline phone for hours. It was a phone that always needed to be charged, a landline phone you'd have to put back on the base to charge. I had a cell phone, too, but the plan wasn't great. I was working at a multinational company and needed a phone during audit fieldwork. My sisters and Mom were annoyed with the phone monopoly I placed on them. At least we had a second line by then, so you could hear the beep when someone else was trying to call.

Darrell and I would play *Yahoo!* pool—never a day missed other than one day when we didn't get to talk. That one day was when he went to visit his friends in another city, and I had a small come apart because he didn't call me that day. Some women do that. We don't mind us going out to visit girlfriends and having a night out often, but when our man does that it gets under our skin – it is maybe insecurity that creeps in. I train myself not to get jealous of Darrell's time with his friends anymore.

What did Darrell and I talk about all those long hours? Food. Certainly not what my aunts thought we talked about. They would pry. "Have you both figured out how many kids you will have?" Good Lord! Heck no. We didn't talk about that kind of stuff. But I was too polite to say that to my aunts. I'd just giggle and redirect the conversation. For Darrell and me, it was all about food. The conversation was, "What did you eat? Was it good? What will you eat next?" It was just comforting to have someone on the other side, even if it was silence on the phone the majority of the time for eight hours on the weekends and four hours every weeknight. To zone out of the tumultuous coming and going of cousins and making chai for uncles and aunts was priceless, a welcome break.

Darrell had done his master's degree in the US and was a Civil Engineer. I was definitely going to move to the US and become an American, as he was already working and established. I was interning in Vancouver and had taken the full-time position after it was offered upon graduation. I'd worked a brief few months, January to April during busy season, and in May was married. Instead of the Chartered Accounting track, I was going to be on the Certified Public Accountant track.

My sister was excited about her wedding day and adding all the bells and whistles she could. She had the fancy henna done. I had the five-dollar not so refined non-bridal henna done. I opted for that. I wanted to save as much money as possible. I figured the weddings were already a huge expense for Mom. I kept telling Mom I was looking to the life beyond, not so much the wedding. I told her repeatedly not to spend on this or that. I wasn't a henna fan anyways; let's skip it altogether. She wasn't having that. I kept telling her to cut the guest list drastically to just family and my close friends. She wasn't having that either. It made her heart very happy though when I told her it wasn't about the wedding for me, it was about moving to the next stage that I was looking forward to.

I was happily anticipating a new start. I looked back at the mountain that went steeply right into the ocean from the fortieth-floor of the downtown company office as twilight was setting in. The view was amazing, and the office was a modern work of art. The office was very well thought out, the corner offices were in fact open bullpens for third year seniors to sit in, not partners, so that everyone can at some point experience a corner office. The sun was setting, but I saw memories there in the distance, of parties downtown, of taking refuge in a junkyard trailer and dark, cold hospitals. Life would be better elsewhere. It was always rainy here anyways, and the winters sometimes would go by with forty days of no sunshine and only gray skies. It was reported that a disproportionately large amount of people in Seattle and Vancouver, which are only 140 miles apart, were on antidepressants.

I was always frugal with Mom's cash – and continued to be during my wedding preparation time. In the first couple years of college my little bit of part-time income from daycares and retail shops would continue to fund my bus fare and my hidden cigarette habit. That hidden nicotine habit followed me, which wasn't easy as my husband also smoked, and culturally women weren't supposed to. He'd be shocked; his family would think only the worst of me. I had to keep it hidden.

Marriage was off to a great start; we bonded quickly. Darrell and I lived in an East Coast town. He moved us out of the garden-level apartment that I felt was so dank and dark, but I never complained about it, except the spiders. Those huge, fuzzy black spiders you notice while sitting on the toilet and make you immobile and petrified. We moved into a second-floor apartment which was amongst greenery and pasture lands. It was a surreal and peaceful setting.

    I had requested my Vancouver office of the multinational company to transfer me to their US office in Darrell's East Coast town; however, there weren't any openings. After moving to the US and about a month in, a position became available. I received a call from the local office of this multinational firm to come in for an interview. The office was on the second floor in a rusty part of downtown, and the people were very antiquated in their philosophies. I made no friends.

    Vancouver was very cosmopolitan and diverse. However this East Coast town was twenty years behind the times. On the West Coast, people dressed very corporate, like it was some sort of competition to look like a celebrity in a magazine. It was Hollywood level. The sophistication in speech, jokes and wit resonated in everyone – it was a big city vibe. Above all it was open-minded. But that was not the case in this much smaller town. People wore ugly shoes and ugly sweaters here, and made homophobic jokes. The people in this office were very catty. One of the downsides of audit world is you are working in smaller groups or just couplets of two professionals in an enclosed client conference room; and it builds the ideal atmosphere for vicious gossip. For hours you fill the time multitasking, working, and listening to the gossip of peers. One day you are sitting with a group where the people are singing praises of one another and overtly cordial with each other during a lunch out. The next day you see those same people back-biting the ones not present from the day before. It was an incessant amount of gossip and malicious behavior in this new office. I'm sure office gossip existed in Vancouver too, and an awful lot of politics in such a large office, but people were much more discreet and careful about it. Maybe in the smaller office people felt they could trust most everyone, and maybe in the bigger office people had learned to not trust anyone.

Compounded with this unease, my medicines were off in this new environment. I had called the employee assistance program (EAP), as acclimating to a new marriage, new city, and new country and having no girlfriends was difficult. Darrell had a very small circle, as he just worked there, hadn't grown up there, and had no major church affiliations or social network either. He was a solitary creature too, like some men are. Perhaps it was the ancestral wiring of the hunter-gatherer societies. It is the theory that men would hunt and become solitary by nature, as opposed to women who would gather supplies and congregate together frequently, becoming wired for that social interaction and connection. He could easily be fine not seeing anyone for a long time, other than me. He always wanted me by his side. My company never bothered him; he craved it. He told me "You're all I need" when I tried convincing him to meet up with various couples from church.

It was lonely for me however, leaving behind a multitude of cousins and friends. After all the lower mainland had been a metropolis of immigrants. I had twenty-plus female cousins in the same city, from both Mom's and Dad's sides. Dad's siblings were all in the lower mainland for decades and still there. Three of Mom's siblings settled there as well. Then there were the work friends from the glitzy and glamorous downtown office of four hundred people. I also had two friends from early high school I had kept in touch with, from that first group of misfits who really were in my corner.

My husband was the kind of man I'd never seen before. He never hit; he never yelled. I was used to problems; I was creating problems. I winced one time, when he raised an arm while talking, thinking he was going to hit me, a blow was coming, and my head jerked and eyes closed.

He asked, "What happened?"

I said, "Oh, nothing. Um, nothing." I never told him what was on my mind. I never told him I thought he was going to hit me.

He shared everything with me, financially, his thoughts, his time; we were true equals and very much each other's other half.

Back home I had only ever heard of relationships where the wife is fairly illiterate and the husband treats her badly and controls everything. A man would never consult on large decisions with his wife, but instead a man will talk to his brother or father or male cousin about a car or land purchase. That's what I saw; women were shut out and barefoot, pregnant, and in the kitchen. The women were fairly abrasive as well, some of them emotionally and verbally abusive, and most all of them confiding in each other as a sorority but never confiding wholly in their men. It creates a mistrust atmosphere and interference in marriages. It's not a marriage of two anymore; it becomes a marriage of many intermingled other female voices building a collage of misunderstanding. Although friends and family are well meaning, they cannot fix a marital problem the way the couple can without that noisy interference.

It's also hard for a spouse to come live in a city where there are a multitude of in-laws and no one of his or her own. That person needs space; the couple needs space. I've heard of many a marriage that broke up, and the pattern is often this set of difficult circumstances.

In the first year, Darrell was controlling I felt, but it took a long time for me to realize I'd misinterpreted the facts and situations due to my own bias and insecurities. I had opened my own bank account, and he was shocked. It was the first time I saw a tear roll down his cheek. I closed the account. The EAP lady suggested it when I called the employee assistance program at work and talked to a therapist. She said, "Have your own finances. It will help you feel independent and in control." I had never paid my mom's bills or written a check other than in accounting class, learning just the theory of it. Mom had done all that. Because Darrell was so much more knowledgeable and experienced, it felt like he was domineering, dictating, and impatient. I was already having work troubles and emotional changes in a new environment. So I processed what the EAP lady told me and went to the bank.

But over the years, I learned from the ten jobs I'd lost—I'd resigned from another two—that each time this identity loss and subsequent insecurity became my hallmark issue where I needed some reassurance on my worth and thus the push for independent finances from Darrell. The loss affected my identity, and I became a complete adversary to him. That happens with spouses; you bear the brunt of each other's animosity. Not the kids or your parents but your other half more often than not becomes the target.

Darrell was a smoker; I hid my addiction from him for about nine months. I'd sneak his smokes when he went to the bathroom. I'd go out on the patio and quickly take some drags. He'd joke, "Hey, are you smoking mine?" when he saw missing ones. He would have never guessed it was the reality though.

He never thought or imagined it because it was so taboo for women to smoke in our culture. Finally, I had to tell him, I needed his help. I had a come to Jesus with him, and he was disappointed for a day. We made up, and then it was easier. I quit finally after what was an eight year smoking stretch. I quit in the busy season of that following year after marriage. However I was still plagued by the fear of that old adage: Once a smoker always a smoker. Physical nicotine withdrawal typically lasts three days as that is the duration for nicotine to clear the system as I understand it. But the mental withdrawal is another matter. On top of this mental willpower challenge, I was about to digress into stark moodiness that was simply a product of me not being able to pay attention enough during an oncoming bout of depression. I had accidently mismanaged my medicines shortly after quitting smoking; something that was purely avoidable and that earned me the animosity of my new work group.

Chapter 11

Postpartum and Fired

2004

A year or so before I had my daughter Madison I switched from the audit practice to the tax department. They had promoted me from a first-year staffer to a second-year staffer upon my arrival to the US office from Canada.

It was a classic mistake of a promotion via a change in company versus earning it through merit and for someone with a weak balance sheet to begin with it is all the more precarious. But I was elated. I'd just been promoted. Years later I was told by HR they had mistakenly understood me to be an In-Charge, and hadn't realized I was an intern for the majority of my Canadian work experience. There had been miscommunication on the level I was at from the former office. This set me up to fail miserably, and I was too timid as someone fresh out of college to anticipate the issues that would occur when expectations are too high and to ask for a demotion.

During my audit time after quitting smoking I was already dealing with my own moodiness, hot and cold toward the staff. Ironically it wasn't because of withdrawal from smoking but rather a dosage change in medication I had done incorrectly. I despised the majority of my colleagues, as they were too different than the corporate family in Vancouver, the family I had went on several week long corporate retreats with over the years and a place where I had bonded with the eleven first years I had shared a first day with.

But I should have had more empathy for my new work family; it was partly me not being open-minded enough. Some people grow up in this small environment, and they are what they are because of their own fears or lack of knowledge. Then there was the additional matter of my medications being off. One Christmas we couldn't go anywhere due to bad weather. I was briefly depressed, and my doctor adjusted my mood stabilizer to double it. I accidently took double the pills at this new higher dose, effectively quadrupling the original dose. I had not paid attention to the fact that the dosage had already been revised and I was to stick with the same number of tablets. I kept popping two of them from the newly prescribed bottle. As a result at work I was feeling like lead and pipes, just cold and devoid of emotion. I was downright mean to coworkers, also very irritable and even almost comatose at times. After a month I realized I was taking the medicines wrong.

I self corrected my erroneously taken medication dosage and got back on track but not before burning bridges with a few individuals on the audit side during my overly medicated time. I became more fodder for office gossip no doubt. I transferred to tax. I could be in the office everyday that way, and with a possibly more amicable and less-back biting set of colleagues. The tax people were close knit and the continuous in office daily interaction allowed for friendships and bonds of camaraderie to develop amongst them.

In audit I was on the road and traveling five weeks straight in busy season. I was going to small predominantly white and low literacy towns where they look at you confused; they'd never seen a brown person I wager. We would often go to audit the local county offices around the state, Yellow Book stuff they called it. It wore on you, the travel.

The locals were awkward but maybe just a bit mystified. One county official would later say of me to the team, as they relayed the message. He asked, "Where is that foreign goddess this time? She didn't come back with you?"

But to me I thought the locals stared rudely. I felt like saying, "The British left the subcontinent decades ago. Brown people are free. Don't look so surprised I'm here." Was it racism or were they just curious?

That was the feel of the audit department in this new East Coast office. Transitioning over to the tax department, there were a different set of challenges. They couldn't tell a pregnant lady like me what she was doing wrong. So it made sense to sweep it under the rug all year, tell her she's doing a great job, and pen the negative feedback on her annual review so you won't have to look at her when you tell her she's doing a horrible job. I made repetitive process mistakes and tax form errors. These were basic things I was missing. I was put on a probationary period, a PIP they call it—performance improvement plan.

The tax partner was beside himself when I told him that it was a complete shock to me; I was never told. I had always been told I was doing a good job. I had driven the long drive back from a vacation I cut short when I received the annual evaluation in my email while out of office. I was a six-month pregnant woman driving alone a full day and left my husband there insisting to him that I had to go in and see the partner immediately. I could think of nothing else. I told Darrell to continue his stay and not worry about me. Internally I felt like that evaluation was enough stress to push me into early labor, so I tried staying calm. My face was flushed the entire drive back. The tax managers and seniors had always kept telling me, "You're doing a good job," and sugarcoating my progress. I was given review notes, but I couldn't read between the lines. I was always book smart not street smart. Natural aptitude and interpreting the grey area was never my strong point, or even something I achieved with mediocrity. I was a linear thinker that took things at face value.

So the PIP was there. I had to fix things fast, or I would be fired, after probation ended. There was certainly no raise. I had already started off with this company at $39,000 USD, and I was stuck at $40,000. I had done poorly in audit. With that department there had been very little raise as I had done poorly there too, drowning in the expectations of the more senior role they had misperceived I was in previously. I was going to deliver my first baby in a few months and utterly stressed. I never negotiated a higher salary with the company when arriving in the US. Darrell told me to, but I figured they'd tell me to go fly a kite if I asked for more. I already had felt stupid at the Vancouver job. I was a team player, but beyond that I was mostly in the mail room photocopying financial documents and doing inventory counts. I wasn't the strongest player there, far from it. There wasn't a good mentor in Vancouver to really be candid with me on where my learning points needed to be; I didn't find a sound straight forward mentor until later in my accounting career. However there was the following conversation I had with a tax manager that was the first glance at an effective mentor conversation… after I was given the PIP this tax manager decided to talk to me in easy terms, which profoundly changed the pace of my work at this small town firm. It was well-placed feedback. He told me he had stuck up for me in the managers' evaluation meeting, an annual meeting that I'd heard over the years would become a witch hunt for staff. He said he told everyone, "Alayna was just starting to break through in audit and get it, and she feels like she needs to do the forms and all the research, and she's failing at trying to do it all." He gave me this anecdotal career-changing advice for tax preparers. "Alayna, you are applying yourself just not in the right way. You have to focus on just getting the forms to look like prior year, and that all boxes are checked in the same manner, and the numbers are coming through and tying. The rest will come later."

Those words were all that it took. I skyrocketed from there with performance. It all fell into place, no more review comments that were process-driven issues. That tax senior is now a Multinational company partner. You only meet a few good mentors in your career, and sometimes you come across none at all. He had said some transparent and straight forward words that made sense to me. Perhaps he was too timid to say them before and maybe he had been coached subsequently, in the aftermath of the partner learning his team had not been giving real time feedback. Some people don't need mentors; they get it out of the gate. Others need more coaching.

 I had my baby girl, Maddy, who I had planned for after the corporation's extended tax due date, which is September 15th of each year. Thankfully Darrell and I had no fertility issues. We picked the days to conceive, and it happened. My contractions started at 12:00 p.m. while at my desk and were two hours apart, and I drove myself home at 3:00 p.m. My colleagues had said, "You're leaving? We can drive you." But I insisted. I was fine.

 It ended up being close to a nineteen-hour labor. The nurses said, "Let's give you some pain medicine," but I had heard in pregnancy class—the one that insurance covered—that it could put the baby to sleep and slow the delivery. I wanted a natural birth. But the baby's heart rate started to dive when contractions happened, a fact found after they strapped on a monitor. I was only three centimeters dilated and cold, clammy, in pain, and finally crying. My husband was with me the whole time, and he told them at 4:00 a.m. I would only start crying if it was really bad. They strapped the monitor around my belly that measured fetal heart rate, and the nurses called in the doctor at 5:00 a.m. She did a C-section around 6:30 a.m. It was one of those left-right incisions, not an emergency up-and-down one thankfully. I have heard the latter type of incision is horrendous afterward, in terms of the healing. The umbilical cord was wrapped around Maddy's neck, which was causing the heart rate to dive during contractions. I held my baby girl. I was thankful for the doctor's actions on doing the C-section timely.

 But a nasty thought crept in my head that I regret to this day. My tradition and upbringing had wired me to feel I should have a boy to make everyone happy. What if my husband was disappointed, like my father was when I was born? Get that thought out of your mind, shame on you, Alayna. My husband was in tears I was told later; he was so happy. Years afterwards I understood the sick conditioning we go through as women of the subcontinent. All mothers love their children and want to keep them. It's the societal and family pressure that causes so much guilt and shame of bearing a female child. Sometimes there is a subsequent abortion propelled forward just by the fact that it is a girl. Not just sometimes I should say, but almost all the time in some parts of the world. There was a wave of abortions in India when this service became available more easily. Decades later, rural India is reeling from not enough girls in the population. With forced wife sharing, some rural Indian areas are getting by in this horrid manner, a problem they didn't anticipate twenty years earlier when all those unborn females were aborted. Sometimes we need to think like economists for most decisions; "where will we be with this decision twenty years from now?"

It was hard to forgive myself for that nasty thought of disappointment when I saw Maddy the first time. I wish I hadn't been conditioned that way or at least recognized where I got the sick thought from and I wish I had pushed it out of the forefront of my mind before it even lingered there for a split second. Where this thought had come from I now realize was the precedent set by Dad and Grandma Edna who at one point had both expressed their disappointment in Mom having only girls. This disappointment they expressed to us girls at an early age had demented us in a certain way to have these regretful thoughts become the default in our mind about our own children. I'm still ashamed somewhat but I understand myself now and what caused that thought. I am gravely apologetic for having that thought after birthing. My mind was still deformed from the decades of backwards cultural conditioning. You should take the best of any culture, not its worst.

During my maternity leave with Maddy I learned I received a midyear raise that increased me to $45,000 even. The local office had approved it with regional, and regional indeed had questioned it greatly, I heard later. "Why? Someone who was on a PIP is now getting a 12.5% raise?" was the argumentative response from the powers that be.

My work performance was good before maternity leave. I went back after eight weeks as that was the only length of maternity leave available at that time. It would have been even shorter at six weeks if it had been a natural birth. But after I went back to work the postpartum manic phase had hit. Most people have heard of postpartum depression. For me it was mania instead.

Winter came, then spring, and the days became longer and markedly brighter earlier, and my sleep was affected. My nanny who I had kept for a few months and who had made my commute easier had to be let go. She was leaving Maddy in her jumping equipment all day. I surprise visited once, and a family friend who flew in from Vancouver also did the same. Both times we found the nanny on the other side of our house on the phone and Maddy alone in her equipment.

Darrell and I decided we needed the grandparents as trusted caregivers. Darrell's parents came into town that spring and moved into their own living space within the same city after living with us initially. They craved their own place. Our home wasn't huge. And they respected our privacy and valued their privacy as well. By April I was driving Madison to Bethany's house across the toll bridge, driving to work, then back to get my daughter, and then back home across town. I was up most nights with infant Maddy as is typical with that stage. My sister Delilah had her second child, a baby boy recently as well. My nephew was going through some health issues, and I flew to the West Coast with Maddy to visit. There was jet lag I hadn't anticipated while already low on sleep taking care of Maddy; it was a dangerous concoction of circumstances for a first time mom with bipolar disorder.

Compounded on these stressors were my sister Emilia's issues she brought me in the know on. Emilia was having guy problems, which I was supposed to keep a secret from Delilah and Mom who were much more traditional than me. Those secrets weighed on me. Emilia's matters fed into my already developing manic frenzy. Additionally the bad memories came back while in Vancouver. As soon as I landed I cried silently when I saw the mountains. They were flooding in, those horrid memories and all that I had left behind in my past life came rushing back as I held Maddy.

My mom wanted me to visit many of her friends and family. There were dinners and lunches lined up. Brown folks persist in that way. It's an Eastern societal norm when you visit, and everyone feels offended if you don't visit them or invite them over. Keeping up appearances was important to Mom. Sometimes the "What will people say?" became a major thing to her.

It was stressful, trying not to be overly chatty, while Mom and Delilah looked over at me with concern at a party. Then coming back to Mom's and having tears set me off on even a glance at an old photo on the shelf. I had rearranged the furniture and strung up the money plant in a beautiful manner by day two; it was looking like a jungle earlier, and now it looked elegant. At first my mom raved at how I had rejuvenated the place, but then she started to notice the energy was manic. My mom gave me sleep medicines, but they did not work.

I flew back after a week in Vancouver and was full-blown manic. I still went to work on Monday after that Sunday flight in. My coworkers could tell I wasn't normal. I was aggressive toward Bethany who always had the kindest heart towards me. I was difficult with Darrell but also elated and euphoric at the same time. He came to get me from work by 11:00 a.m. on Tuesday.

The medicines were slow to work; my psychiatrist at the time didn't understand I needed heavy sleep medicines immediately upon the onset of a manic phase. She had long before asked me if I was okay to talk with students in her field as I was fascinatingly a high functioning person with bipolar disorder.

But for confidentiality reasons I declined. With this episode, she decided to do a slow increase of my antipsychotic and mood stabilizer dosage together with adding an anti-anxiety medicine for relaxation and sleep. That was the frustratingly slow way to do it though and wasn't effective for me in nipping it in the bud but rather making it a five month recovery process and the mania would come back one more time in that timeframe. Unless I had a hospital injection or took three of the five insomnia medicines I had later in life, it was going to be a slow, painful process to get back to normal. The family had to deal with my erratic behavior for an unnecessarily long and drawn out time due to medicines that were not strong enough. I told my husband I didn't want to go to the hospital, and neither could he ever think of putting me there. For me being able to sleep 10+ hours initially would have greatly helped the recovery process but I went from a half hour of sleep nightly to maybe four hours at most after her dosage change.

I took a month of FMLA disability leave that entire May. When I came back to work in June, the local office really wanted me to be transparent with them and tell them what was going on. The tax partner gave me every opportunity to tell him without being invasive about it. But I was scared. Years later I realized they only wanted to help. But at that time, I didn't want to lose my job. Maybe if I could tell them I had bipolar, they would cut me some slack. But I thought to myself, I'd be fired the next major mistake I made. Who wants instability in the workplace sitting next to them or working for them? To this day, of all my jobs I've had, I'm not sure telling any Human Resource (HR) departments or bosses would be a good thing for me.

I'm going to pause here and mention that people face many mental health challenges in the workplace and larger companies are trailblazing the initiative to recognize this. The below is inserted from the *National Alliance on Mental Illness's* website:

Even though so many people face mental health challenges in the workplace and at home, negative stereotypes still exist. These stereotypes and misconceptions are called stigma. Together, we can all

do our part in helping American workplaces thrive by ridding them of stigma. Mental health is everyone's concern and its consequences to the workplace in particular are tremendous:
- Mental health conditions are the leading cause of disability across the United States.
- Untreated mental health conditions cost the economy $200 billion in lost earnings each year through decreased work performance and productivity.
- 8 of 10 workers with a mental health condition report that shame and stigma prevent them from seeking treatment.
- The family is also affected, increasing the use of leave time for family members.

StigmaFree Company is NAMI's partnership initiative to challenge, highlight and cultivate a company culture of caring and enhanced engagement around mental health. By being a StigmaFree Company and prioritizing mental health as a workplace and community priority, you will help:
- Increase productivity and promote a healthier work environment;
- Decrease the impact of disability;
- Increase retention and engagement of valued employees; and
- Strengthen your company brand by linking to a cause that resonates with so many.
- What Does A StigmaFree Company Look Like?

Brands and companies have a crucial role to play in the mental health of their employees, customers and consumers as well as communities overall. We need companies' help to raise awareness that mental health conditions are not the result of personal weakness, lack of character or poor upbringing—and that knowing the facts about mental illness can help reject stigmatizing stereotypes.
— www.nami.org

There is hope to continue the dialogue of mental illness and eradicate its stigma at some point in the future and starting this discussion in every workplace is a need now more than ever.

During this manic episode after returning from Vancouver with Maddy, I confided to my husband about the incest I had went through at age ten. I thought my mom would be the only one to ever know of the incest, but here I was at age twenty-five, the information came tumbling out to my husband as well when I was episodic; like it did almost a decade earlier sitting in Delilah's room before I was admitted to the hospital the first time. I wouldn't have told Darrell about the incest if I had stayed episode free. A vault had sealed the knowledge of incest which that perpetrator boy's sister had made sure stayed only in my mind and otherwise would never have been divulged to a soul. I don't think I would have ever planned to tell Darrell about the incest over my life time. No good could come of it I felt. But maybe at some turn I would have realized the burden of the secret was too much, and he would accept it and not be disgusted with it. My Mom I had also only told inadvertently because of being episodic, and history repeated itself again with me confiding the truth to Darrell.

I divulged to my mom later that I had told Darrell about the incest. Mom was mortified that I had told him, she was worried he'd leave me. She didn't understand how much we had bonded already in those first two years. She'd never had a healthy relationship herself to know a man's unconditional love. Darrell was my rock, and I felt comfortable enough with him, but I still wonder when and if I would have told him of the incest had it not come out because of an episode where I was in euphoric mania; one in which I could not remain tight-lipped and I had felt on top of the world. With the decades going by and more solidarity in our marriage I hope there would have been a point in life where I would have told him voluntarily and while completely in my senses. I never got the chance though in life, it was just disclosed in a rambling during this manic episode.

The perpetrators in the extended family who were involved in the incest found out too that they had been uncovered further and to someone outside the family now. I hope shame befell them. They were questioned by their parents even as adults. How can these cousins meet mine or Mom's gaze ever again? I certainly can give them a cutting look though. I remember you, and what you did – that glare would say. They were fiends. Albeit kids themselves at the time of the incident. But still they were old enough to know better. The main perpetrator was sixteen, he was the fondler. He had asked another cousin who was eleven-year-old to expose himself to all the kids in the room. I was the only female there. These actions and memories incriminated me for years in my mind, as victims always feel it is their fault. The victim instigated it somehow; the victim should have done something different. That's how you feel about yourself and it keeps you closed up. The mind is a horrible thing for a person, and even more so for one with bipolar disorder, where your own mind is your biggest enemy already. I do still wonder whether this incest factor was the reason my disorder was activated in my genes.

    I'm at this stable confident stage now in life where I've done far better than any of these boys in life, weathered storms, come through and stood taller than them. They probably never thought I had a chance in life, the daughter of a divorcée, rumored to be a "mental case." She would keep shut and hide herself forever they likely wagered.

    Back in those days – and perhaps even now some Indians didn't understand mental illness. A lot of the illiterate population felt a person with the illness was just an idiotic individual who had messed up thoughts and was a few steps away from being in a straight jacket in an asylum. Some mentally ill Indians are medically treated with drugs but still don't live a fully functional life. I know personally of some sufferers, in other families where word couldn't be kept in, as it was too obvious the person was dealing with a brain imbalance. These individuals are plagued with frequent episodes. Their medicines might not have been discovered for their ideal balance based on the individual, which is a trial-and-error process. Dually with this lack of medication balance, they lack self-awareness to really understand how their illness affects them, their families, and to fully accept what they have. Sometimes the people around them have difficulty separating the illness from the person, taking it as though they have a character defect.

Sometimes the bipolar patient's family has given up and is at the hinge of abandoning them. Abandonment especially if it's a wife or in-law who is clinically depressed, and sponsored into the New World. Often the new atmosphere destabilizes individuals. I've heard cases where they will send an Indian wife back to her family. I've also noticed an Indian husband afflicted with this illness has it two fold worse, as he was to provide for the family. What will the family do now? The wife in that instance sometimes out of frustration doesn't know how to handle it and seeks her kin to help save the marriage. Running also for protection as well, if the husband has violent tendencies that typically become even more amplified with this disease of the brain. Some spouses are doubly frustrated, not understanding what the illness needs. Medicine, but counseling too? Or anger management sessions? They continue with a huge dose of family pain and patience as the children look on at the horrors in the household. The situation is made ten times worse when the sufferer refuses to accept help or to stay on medication.

Perhaps because I became self-aware and didn't stay in denial after my second episode I don't tend to have a lot of sympathy for people with bipolar disorder who stay unaware and deny they have an illness. It is frustrating to learn some don't take medicines intentionally – they refuse to listen to the concerns of their loved ones. There are those who are born into homelessness or have parents that were direly ill themselves or abusive, for those I understand never attaining stability or self awareness and acceptance of your condition. But for everyone else if life gave you a chance at stability, you have a huge step up to manage this illness with the help of a loved one or your own self awareness and setting up of support systems while fully in your own on a proactive basis. Self-pity is a terrible thing to fall into and try to find comfort in. I feel like the self pity can quickly consume your ownership of trying to keep yourself mindful, present and aware.

The person with bipolar disorder needs love and understanding. They are not bipolar; they have bipolar disorder. Some would treat a diabetic relative who has an insulin deficiency with respect. A mentally ill relative with a lithium deficiency in the brain may have a whole different judgment placed on them by the same people.

Darrell would give me my medicines and I would giggle at this, and take the new doses prescribed to nip the Vancouver trip's mania. These medicines I thought were part of some sort of game where people were secretly watching us in our home via satellite monitoring and surveillance and expected us to play along via subtle communications. But then Darrell got very serious, and asked me pointedly what was so funny. Immediately I was embarrassed and realized this was not a game. I realized the utter desperation in his voice. I am embarrassing myself again with this illness I thought. In my mind's eye I then recalled my previous episode when I was completely out of it at a party with about a hundred people where similar regrets of embarrassing behavior lingered forever in memory. I realized then and there this is a real problem. Darrell was gravely concerned, I could finally see it in his eyes when my delusions of conspiracy around us faded with his comment to stop laughing and that there was nothing funny about any of this. I was on leave for four weeks but the doctor's note expired after that and I was set to go back to work. I went back to work that first week of June but wasn't entirely in my own still. Darrell and I realized later that four weeks is not enough time to resituate from mania – it's a direct function of how long I've gone sleepless for. In the Vancouver trip case it must have been over a week of insomnia.

About a month passed while back at work, and June rolled to an end. I hadn't truly recovered. I couldn't focus with the mania still not entirely cured and it was starting to come back. My medicines hadn't given me my true eight to nine hours sleep that

I was normally sleeping. I had seemed fine at the surface level to go back to work, at least in my own mind and then Darrell felt I was fine as well. We didn't want to chance being away very long and lose the job. It was his first rodeo with the illness, so he didn't recognize there maybe something still lurking under the bipolar waters. The psychiatrist had only written for four weeks of leave to begin with and didn't extend it as I seemed functional enough after the meeting with her during the end of that time span. This doctor really didn't have a good read on me or to ask any of the right questions – perhaps I'm asking too much of any doctor that sees you for only a half hour. Perhaps she just wasn't perceptive enough and didn't have experience with a high-functioning bipolar person who can appear fine but isn't. I was so immensely frustrated with what happened next. If I had just been out longer, it would have been okay. I may still have had my Multinational company job.

Not until Hudson did I realize that it takes about four months of downtime to regain your judgment 100 percent from a full blown manic episode, one in which you haven't slept three days straight at least. Darrell already knew to a degree when this hit a second time that a month wouldn't be enough and to make sure I stayed away for the workplace longer.

At the Multinational company in early July, I sent an email I had worked on overnight on my home computer. I thought people would love it, and it would be hilarious. I sent it to the 'All Employees' email group and additionally copied the regional office. My judgment was shot by then. The email was meant to be light and humorous in my episodic mind but was taken as mean-spirited and discriminatory. It was sent on a Monday. Regional called local and said, "You need to fire her. This email could be seen as discriminatory." HR liabilities were high in this case. Regional wouldn't hear of keeping me although the local office had told them I had been out on leave for something likely related to a mental health issue. The home office knew I had recently been on disability and erratic. On Tuesday the tax partner called me into his corner office, and the

HR director was already seated there. The paperwork was on the desk in front of me. I signed it immediately, not in my right mind. I was being terminated for a discriminatory email.

The HR director lady said, "You have a work visa; we are required to give you a ticket home."

I said, "No, my family is here." I started crying and was walked out with a box of my belongings and family pictures in hand.

The tax partner's hands were tied. I'd sent the email to regional as well. Had it stayed in the home office, they could have handled it. He told me that two weeks later when I called him, pleading for my job back, by then I had also asked the doctor to send him a note explaining the situation which the doctor had done. He had told me he had given me many chances to tell them if there was something wrong, and that they could have helped more but I had remained silent. He said it was out of their hands now because I had copied regional otherwise they would have handled it in their office. I wager if they had known I was dealing with a mental illness they could have immediately deflected regional headquarters demand to fire me and the illness diagnosis would have resonated with the powers above and the matter written off for some mandatory time off and additional diversity training. The company was one of the largest in the world and local HR was not made privy to why someone was on disability unless the worker told them directly – the privacy was protected and my doctor and Darrell had faxed the disability letter back in the beginning of May based on the company's process to the Out of State headquarters for disability claims. My team was concerned for months already, and I was never forthcoming with them on what I was really going through. They only could speculate from my erratic behavior that there was something I might be dealing with. They never knew for sure, and then that behavior became overtly worse manifesting itself in an email sent to everyone in the office and beyond just local. Regional took that step of requiring termination. Perhaps if the issue had stayed at local and no one else outside the local office had gotten wind of that email there would have been more remorse and control over the termination decision.

Even with summer's brightness and persistent sun I became depressed. Counseling would have been great. I kept dumping my negativity onto Bethany and her husband, both had moved back in to help take care of Maddy and me as well, since I was suffering from depression now as losing a prestigious job blew out all of my confidence and deflated me entirely. I was given stronger medicines. I was starting to sprout thick neck hair as a result of some of these new medications. I kept calling the nurses' phone line and trying to talk to them for reassurance and guidance. They said, "We can't treat you over the phone. Make an appointment, and counseling sessions run ninety dollars a session." Insurance didn't cover much of those fees at all.

Darrell said, "Go for a few sessions. Just do it. It will make you feel better. Don't worry about the expense." I couldn't think of spending that kind of money. Darrell would be disappointed too I felt inside. He was working hard and broken over a nonfunctional wife with an illness he barely knew anything about and a child that remained neglected by her completely, Bethany was solely handling Maddy at this stage of my depression. Maddy went to the West Coast with her grandparents to their daughter's house so they could have help taking care of their granddaughter for a month while I tried to regain my mental balance.

Bethany was exhausted by then and needed her daughter's help. I was still very depressed the two months after losing my job. Bethany was worried though without Maddy I may fall into further depression. But I was so detached from the world I barely acknowledged her most of the time. It was a sad state, literally.

When it was just Darrell and I again, he would take us out to fast-food and sit-down restaurants, but I'd stare into space. Finally, one day a smile broke on my face with laughter. Darrell smiled, too, and stared at me in a hopeful way. He hadn't smiled in a long time either. I caught an episode of *Star Trek - The Next*

Generation on TV. There was a comical scene with Data, the android, which made me laugh. I had grown up watching this series, so the show had nostalgic value for me.

During this third episode, I was suicidal. It was the only episode I had seriously considered ending my life. Losing the Multinational company accounting job was too much for me to handle. It had been an enviable job for five years, starting in the Canadian office and ending here in the US. This job and company name was my identity. Mania had worn off almost immediately after the job loss and suddenly there was no more office work or commute and 50 hours of additional time suddenly freed up. Now I was at home and expected to take over domestic tasks and child rearing entirely, and depression hit.

The suicidal thoughts went as such: I played it over in my mind, going to the shed in the night when all were asleep, where Darrell stored his tools and the snow blower. I would use the chain saw or something; it would be quick. These thoughts plagued me, especially at night. They hounded me when I was alone with my thoughts, lying next to a sleeping Darrell. These thoughts slowly became less frequent as I normalized and found the middle of the sinusoidal curve – that middle area between depression and mania, where one reaches a mentally balanced equilibrium.

I had run into suicidal individuals in the lockdown wards years earlier. I always looked down upon them. I was, for the most part, never one of them. I was too elated in mania and too happy to even think about harming myself or anyone else. But now I understood depression, and I have remorse for those individuals – I can still vividly picture the despair in their eyes as I lived through that myself during this postpartum time. Bethany would say my name at times to bring me back to the present as I sat across the room from her, because I'd be staring into space otherwise. An empty mind can become the devil's den and she sensed it wasn't good for me to be so quiet.

Jobless and in the US now, I realized I had to be in this country legally. Darrell knew about the immigration rules and told me it would be fairly serious being here long term without the proper status. I had to find another job as soon as possible. He was still a green card holder and had put in my sponsorship application but it was a very long process that would take years for formal approval. So I had to be in the US on the grounds of work status to make staying legal, otherwise staying as simply a Canadian visitor wasn't in the cards because I had an active spousal sponsorship application in process and technically had to be waiting in my home country for US approval to arrive legitimately. The only grounds to stay in the US during a spousal sponsorship waiting period were if I had an alternate status in tandem such as an active work visa.

During the time Maddy was on the west coast I started interviewing after I came out of my reverie and commenced corresponding again with Darrell in a more engaged manner. A local giant CPA firm hired me through a recruiter, who put an awful lot of spin on my résumé. I had Multinational company experience, but why was I only paid $45,000 so many years into it? The recruiters were perplexed only for a second; they immediately knew I likely had performance issues. They also instantly must have realized I had been let go from the previous job. When they asked why I was no longer there I had just said "I left for medical reasons" as the explanation. They couldn't pry more than that. The recruiters had recruitment fees to earn so they pushed me in front of this company. They were pushing a square peg into a round hole. I wasn't ready for a senior role still – I had just started doing well in tax for a few months around the time of Maddy's birth. I was probably just the equivalent of a first year tax staff, but my salary climbed to $55,000 in the Senior role. Darrell was congratulatory to me, but I was cringing at the expectation and responsibility. I went back to smoking.

Bethany, Maddy and her grandpa came back to our home and Darrell went to another city for a new higher-paying job. I knew I was only going to be at the local firm for another two months before I left. When I resigned from there, the managing partner refused to shake my hand at the exit interview when I had extended it to him as farewell. He said I'd cost him all these filing fees for the work visa and he stormed out of the office leaving me with the HR administrator. I had to reimburse them part of the legal fees as I was leaving them early; they had sunk a couple thousand into my visa application on their end also. They let me go even before my two weeks notice period was up. It was after the October 15th extended deadline for when individual taxes had passed, and I was shown the door soon after putting in my two week resignation. There wasn't much work to be done at that time of year anyways. The managing partner was irate about the expensive recruiter fee they had incurred also. I'm hoping there was something in their contract to say the candidate has to stay a certain amount of months otherwise the recruiting fee is refunded back. I felt awfully guilty using them for legitimate work status temporarily. It's just business a shrewd mind would say though.

My husband was a green card holder at this time, not a citizen yet, so my sponsorship was slow and lower priority. So I had a work visa, and that was my grounds to be in the US legally. I had to keep continuous employment. As a Canadian you can only visit for six months at a time otherwise. Luckily I had accepted a position in the new city before handing in my resignation so it wasn't as daunting to be unemployed again as this time it was temporary.

Bethany had taken care of Maddy for months now and Maddy was attached to her very much but Bethany always told me that mom is mom and Maddy needs me. She would tell me Maddy doesn't light up the same way when she sees her as she does when she sees me. Bethany encouraged me to pay attention to her. It was hard though, I was groggy always because of the medicines, one of them was entirely new, not just an enhanced dose of something I'd already been taking. It was a blood pressure medicine that I was to take four times a day and was supposed to help the mind stabilize. The two month job was an interesting one where I had to hide taking pills at least twice daily while at work.

Bethany was a blessing as I didn't want Mom to come help during this episode. I was so full of anger at my childhood and blaming her for its darkness. It took years to feel better about her again. I regret to this day I shut Mom out.

Bethany was there as the second mom I really needed – and she helped manage the household while I worked in this new temporary job before we could move to the other city Darrell had moved to for work. During my depression, Darrell had some leave from work but had to go back eventually – and during this time he figured he'd look for something better. At the edge of his mind he realized it would be up to him solely to financially support us at times in life so he needed to earn proportionately more than when it was the two of us earning together.

This was the first his family had seen of bipolar disorder up close. It is even harder for the family trying to manage the loved one with bipolar disorder. The bipolar disorder individual is euphoric, everything is fine, and we live with the guilt afterward of our actions and what we put people through. The loved ones actually live it and survive and suffer through it in an even more acutely trapped manner.

I take a detached view of what is happening when episodic where I know I am hurting my loved ones and I can see the worry is killing them inside but I cannot stop myself from the erratic behavior. There is a perception and awareness that exists during this phase when you are not in your own; but you continue with the behavior because the thoughts rapidly race and focus doesn't stay on any particular, even remotely rational, thought. Many regrets of what was said and done linger afterwards for a lifetime.

Darrell had earned many promotions and excelled at what he did with the company he'd worked for ten years already on the east coast. He had several offers from larger cities both on the East Coast and in the Midwest, and we decided on the Midwest one. By this time I'd experienced the West Coast and East Coast but not the Heartland. Finally October arrived and we could move westward and be together as a family again.

    Around these years there were some realizations I'd made. As I experienced life as a mother for the first time I would often recall what should have been better mothering of my younger sister who Delilah and I looked after. For my younger sister, Emilia, I have my regrets with how I treated her. Delilah and I raised our little sister while Mom was at work, making ends meet, shift work that would last till store closing where she would get back home at 1:00 AM from the fast food restaurant.
    We were kids, ourselves. I was snarky and mean to Emilia and somewhat manipulative to gain her affection and admiration at times.
    Emilia grew up with Mom giving her the bank debit card as a show of love because there was no bandwidth on Mom's end to spend quality time with her outside of just childcare at times. Emilia went away to college after Delilah and I got married; she was excited to get accepted – and escape the mundane set of cousins in the lower Mainland of which most on my mom's side were fresh off the boat from India. She was annoyed with their nosey, overly traditional, antiquated and meddling tendencies.
    A year in after Emilia's university started, my mom happened to open up a letter in the mail, and it stated that Emilia was on academic probation. She had partied away the twenty thousand dollars my mom had saved up for her room and board and education fees. She hadn't spent that time studying and making the most of Mom's hard-earned money. There was no bonding between mother and daughter over the years, and this was even more obvious as the years progressed. Their relationship evolved into unfortunately a transactional one at best.
    Emilia had never seen how life was as a family with both parents under one roof. She never really missed her dad as she never experienced life with a dad. Delilah and I had seen Mom suffer through separations, abuses, and making ends meet. We were old enough. I was protective of her money, and Delilah

kept the house running. My older sister knew at age fifteen how to cook curries and biryani. Dinner would be ready every night for us younger sisters and a portion set aside for Mom for when she got home. Emilia however never bonded with any of us. At least Delilah and I had seen some memories of happiness in childhood when things were sporadically peaceful between Mom and Dad. But Emilia had never experienced a complete family bonding that was seemingly secure to childhood eyes.

Emilia ran away from home after she had come back that summer and found that her academic probation had been discovered by Mom. She hated the cousins always coming over and the Eastern lifestyle and expectations of looking like a showpiece for possible marital prospects. She left home abruptly. She went back to Alberta and worked in a women's shelter for a few years near an Aboriginal Canadian Reservation where she had emotionally quit from on the spot and then had worked with a Canadian mental health agency, a federal job she couldn't keep either. She also had a plethora of other places she'd worked at between then and 2019. She was like me. She had Mom, and I had Darrell. We had a safety net and didn't take jobs too seriously when the going got tough.

Emilia didn't grow up with a dad in the house the majority of her childhood, just like me, and because of this we both didn't understand authority. She suffers from persistent depressive disorder, I'd guess from my research. I could never bring this research up to her. I brought it up to Mom though. Emilia is now in her early thirties and every now and then has taken antidepressant medication. We always thought her depression was situational or seasonal. Living so far north in Canada, the days are small in winter. It's like Iceland or Scandinavia, where people have bouts of depression often given the extreme sunlight fluctuations and mood at times correlates with seasons. Then the job losses were a situational factor, and life dually became a roller coaster. We lost Emilia many times over to the Prairie Provinces she kept finding work in; she didn't want to come back home.

My mom and Delilah stayed in the same traditional rut for a decade, pressuring Emilia to get married to an Indian man and conform to Indian society.

One year Emilia called the cops on Mom, after Mom had exclaimed, "You can leave, but you're not taking the car I bought for you," an attempt on Mom's end to keep Emilia here – Mom hadn't had a greedy stance at all in fact, it was just a persuasive measure. Emilia was angry at this and dialed 911 (an emergency call). After the cop incident, I didn't talk to her for eight years. I also hadn't seen her in person for a 12 year stretch. She kept losing jobs, and Mom was called as a safety net every time. It was like the Bank of Mom was always open. Delilah and I were frustrated at Emilia always tapping into this bank with no obligation. Emilia would cry over the phone to Mom, and Mom would weaken immediately. Mom would send a wire to Emilia's bank account the same day so Emilia had some cash to survive. That was their transactional relationship from the beginning. Mom didn't have bandwidth for quality time with Emilia during her childhood so bonding with her was difficult. Mom conveyed her affection for Emilia through buying her the things she really wanted. The materialistic wants being fulfilled could never bridge the gap of missing bonding time between mother and daughter.

Emilia would cry when we were talking at times. But I started to see through it as I gained my own wisdom. I told her pointedly, "Emilia, don't play that game with me. People can see through stuff like that." She immediately stopped the emotional manipulation attempts.

Emilia ended up in a homeless shelter once. Delilah told me, but I don't know the details directly – likely after a job loss I'm assuming. She has a fur baby, originally a puppy who was only eight weeks old when she adopted him and that keeps her from going out of her mind; otherwise, she'd be mired in an even deeper depression.

I pray life works out wonderfully for Emilia. She was always our baby. When I say her name, I sometimes say my daughter's name instead and have to correct it. In my mind there is that protection of her and a soft spot. It is bittersweet. Sometimes there is seething hate at what she did and sometimes there is empathy and love as well. Occasionally I have dreams of everything being normal between us two. Like the sisterhood we never had and to start from scratch again.

Fast forward a few years - Emilia was suicidal recently, and her friend had reached out to Delilah and me. I hadn't seen the message but only with great delay as it went to my social media account's secondary inbox. But luckily the friend got a hold of Delilah live.

This friend told Delilah that Emilia was considering suicide. Emilia had lost a job over the previous winter, a sweatshop-type job where she suspected the owner was money laundering from a side drug business. The owner coerced her into staying when she quit on the spot, bullying her by bringing all the workshop men into the office for intimidation. Emilia, this time, battled her boss for severance—three months' worth—and his lawyer drew up paperwork that she would not defame him (in his mind, report his activities) to anyone ever. She signed and had it paid to her. She was worried his checks would bounce. She was deeply anticipating to cash the postdated checks each month – she needed the money badly as she had always been paycheck to paycheck. Delilah at times would draw up a budget for Emilia and encourage her to save. But Emilia had our mom as a safety net always, and my guess is this fact never motivated her to save her own money.

After quitting Emilia had packed up her belongings and rode back in my brother-in-law's (Delilah's husband's) truck. He had driven to Alberta from BC and helped put all her things in the trailer, and drove west to Mom's house fourteen hours away.

This wasn't the first time Emilia was chaperoned by Delilah's husband. In years past, Delilah's husband had ferried her back to her place in Alberta as she wanted to escape the Vancouver life again, and left Mom's affection hanging. During this drive Delilah's husband had somberly told her: "Emilia, if you ever reconcile with your sisters and mom – they will take you back, but I won't, and neither will Darrell, ever accept you back." He cared a great deal for his mother-in-law, he was the son she'd never had. He wanted to somehow move Emilia to say she will stay back in Vancouver and he could turn the truck around to arrive back to a Mom that would be relieved to see her daughter again. But it didn't happen, not that year. Not until a decade later did she return and with the intention of staying.

    Eventually Mom sold both previous homes after long property settlements in the 90s and, after saving up, was able to mortgage a larger property that my sister Delilah devoted her energy to planning the entire custom build. Delilah loved that stuff, even with four kids. She made all those trips to pick out faucets, lights, etc. It was a good escape from baby world for Delilah. She loved interior design. This was Mom's dream house put into brick and mortar reality all with Delilah's help, finally in her 60s Mom was able to afford building her dream house ground up.
    In this large house Mom had foreign exchange students and other renters occupy the rooms so she could continue to pay the mortgage, alongside her fast-food manager's paycheck. But these renters always were a hot mess, leaving dishes piled up for five days at a time in their rooms. That was just one of the problems. Another major problem was their excessive non-judicious amount of laundry that would compound the utility bill. She had a tenant that would do one load for underwear, one for pants, etc. These were ridiculous and ostentatious liberties. Mom was always on the agreeable and pleasant side of the spectrum with her renters. But it wore on her. Finally she would have to evict them one by one based on some fabricated grounds that family was moving in and she needed the additional space.

Chapter 12

Hudson and Another Job Lost

2006

I had five interviews in one day in the new city at various-sized CPA firms; with a Multinational company on your résumé, it is definitely easier to get selected as an interview candidate. At that time I had sent in a physical mail-in copy, not electronically via email. Maybe I wasn't as resourceful to find the right electronic link. So I sent in résumés with signed cover letters in fall of 2006. I was invited to meet with all the companies I had sent résumés into and had two job offers from the five interviews I had all in one day. I took the regional company firm offer instead of the local large firm. The local firm was placing me at a manager level, which made me nervous, but the pay was much more too. I wasn't confident at all in my abilities for that level. The manager position was twenty thousand dollars higher than the other offer.

Darrell didn't understand how I would want to take the lower offer. I told him I didn't think I could survive. At that point I had maybe accumulated a first-year tax staff and first-year audit staff's combined experience. I couldn't see myself going into a manager level abruptly. At the regional company firm I was starting with in this new city, they had already stuffed me one rung higher into a senior position; the manager level would have been an even bigger leap from where I was at now. My work experience had started in 2001 with an internship, then a year in between of school. So effectively I'd already had what looked like five years on my résumé by now.

I had told the recruiter at the regional accounting firm that I wanted to be a tax staffer, not tax senior. She said, "But don't you want to be a senior?" She had a requisition to fill as a recruiter; that was her job. She made it sound like I was a deadbeat and that I really needed to strive harder, or that's how I interpreted it. I fell right into her expectation, being inexperienced and timid. I had already been pushed to second-year staff earlier with the Multinational firm upon arriving in the US. Here I was again in the same situation. I was nervous, and anxiety crept in. Later in my years, I knew my balance sheet and skill set and what I didn't know. I knew what I could and could not do and went into interviews much more confident, assertive, and authoritative, and the whole while diplomatically balanced. But at this stage I wasn't there yet, with the recruiter's pointed question I caved and said anxiously, "Yes, of course, senior is fine".

The two years at this firm was boot camp. I learned a lot. But it was knowledge I couldn't apply and process, because I didn't have the confidence, which I now know is the key factor to success.

I was pregnant with my second child, a boy. I had learned a lot of tax compliance from a tax partner who was like none other. This partner was a tax heavyweight. The gray-haired partners would research something to the nth degree and, stumped on proper tax treatment, would go to his office cube for answers to corroborate their findings, and he'd correct them in one breath on the right treatment without looking at any guidance. He had told me that in his younger days he had read the tax code before work daily, an extra knowledge enhancement the others didn't gain.

Partners sat in cubicles at this company. It was an open office environment. Back then it was very new age and uncommon for a corporate environment to be this way. It was a very organic, decentralized and non-hierarchal culture.

Sometimes I'd cry on the weekends at my desk in frustration on just not getting it. But I was too afraid to ask the tax partner again for help or the tax manager on Monday as I'd look incompetent. I was a senior after all; it was expected I know. If you keep asking the same questions in year three or five of your career, that's a major issue.

I had gone back to smoking a brief few months, before pregnancy, as I was so stressed. The expectations were so incredibly high. I already had a number of years behind me, with the internship starting in the third year of school and then two more work histories from the other US city. It was difficult to dummy down the experience and years on my résumé.

I hadn't ever thought of showing a gap and taking years off. Now with twenty years behind me, I've only shown three employers with longer tenures, not the other nine or so I worked at where I lost most of those jobs anyways.

I've accumulated a wealth of experience, mostly making mistakes not to repeat over again. I've also acquired an infusion of many firms and best practices I can borrow knowledge from. At the current stage I'm a contractor and love it so far. They don't own you eight to five, and you don't need to respond right away to demonstrate you're tethered to your desk and an available employee during most waking hours.

Today, I work from home virtually for a firm in another state. My husband has benefits so I don't need to be an employee, and I'm part time so further not tied to a desk or email or instant messaging system. I'm an independent contractor now. As life happens, with its ups and downs, and office politics and family tragedies, it's hard to sit in a bustling office and behave as a CPA with bipolar disorder. My husband has steadily climbed the ladder, dealing with bad bosses and lots of stress. Without bipolar disorder perhaps it's easier, or men just compartmentalize better; for many they don't bring it to work with them when there is a squabble at home. Some women can compartmentalize; but I can't. I fixate on personal matters at my work desk and cannot push those troubles from my mind so easily. Darrell was offered the VP position recently at work; I'm proud of him. It's a firm of four thousand employees.

I hope I helped make that success possible. Behind every successful man is a woman. I held the household all those years, raised the kids, and struggled to keep jobs but gainfully employed with very minimal downtime most of my career and earning money and continually adding to our savings and retirement – peace of mind for Darrell at least in that regard. I wasn't able to keep a job, but I could find a job quickly after losing one and be earning most of the time.

Had I been a homemaker, maybe those episodes wouldn't have happened though or as severely. I could have slept during the day to ward off jet lag during that one trip where the episode wasn't work related in 2006. The rest of the episodes wouldn't have happened if I wasn't working – they were directly tied to a work event trigger.

Mothering isn't easy to begin with and further complicated for a person with bipolar disorder. In those early years, the kids wake up and come to your room even through age five. Hudson would sleepwalk, which would jerk me awake at night worrying about him. I took the majority of kid responsibilities. Darrell had to be functional for his job. Without his income we'd be a mess. I couldn't be relied on to keep a job anyways. In hindsight had I quit when I got my green card, life would have been less episodic. But you give up some luxuries that way. I managed to gather one million of wages in the last seventeen years in the US based on my social security statement. That makes me feel somewhat accomplished although it was a multitude of jobs. It was helpful to be a part of that building of assets for the family. Now I can drop my load; Darrell understands. At this point in my forties, he just wants me to be happy and not run the rat race I was so bad at running.

As a work-from-home, part-time contractor, I get my work done in a focused, productive manner. There is no water-cooler talk, and no ostentatious meals out at lunch or long car rides with colleagues where you might become loose tongued and say too much in the closeness of the environment. There are no more rich office lunches and vendors bringing in treats to make your battle with the bulge harder. Neither is there a commute that sucks the life out of you and is time wasted that you aren't paid for. Such commute time is one that you can never get back in a day or apply to any meaningful task or self-care time.

It's a blessing to finally try something new. I'm a Generation X person. For Millennials I hear that job hopping is common and acceptable to see on their resume. But for someone with twenty years behind them on their résumé, it can look awfully bad to keep trying new things. I chalk up my years out of work on my résumé to mothering now, knowing full well those years were filled with failed work endeavors. Honestly, I was mothering and handling my job poorly postpartum. So why show the job?

I haven't lied. I didn't add anything on my résumé I didn't do; I took away from it. I included less experience. That, to me, I can do with a straight face in an interview. I am removing the non value-added learning and time. Short stints should be moved off resumes anyways I feel, and I move to a year-to-year format versus a month-year format on the dates employed disclosure so the date gaps don't glare back at a hiring manager.

This date smoothing gets your foot in the door I feel. Once they have talked to you and they like you, that's the paramount deciding factor. You can fill out the application later where the exact dates are stated and gaps are visible. An HR processor may just leave it alone and it won't seem like there is a hidden issue like a firing. I've never been questioned on the gaps after the in-person interview.

I interview very well, charismatic, confident, diplomatic and sociable with well timed and tasteful humor used sparingly. It has been a blessing to quickly land a job at all these bad turns in the past.

By that time the company has met you in person and likes you anyways. But it depends on the company size too on if your gaps will remain unscrutinized. Large companies that have an army devoted to background checks and reviews of applications will dig and question more. But for small and midsize firms my experience has been that it's a bit more relaxed with limited bandwidth for them to deep dive.

I leave those giant gaps of two years each on my résumé now at this current stage of life. I was mothering; I had two kids. The luxury of being a stay-at-home mom (SAHM) simply is how I render the story of those gaps. If only I had actually done that during that time, a SAHM life; perhaps I'd have had more mental stability during the time my family was young. Postpartum is a difficult time for those even without bipolar disorder and to have the illness is a huge compounding factor where something has to give in order to stay on top of what is important during a time when one is most vulnerable to instability.

As related to the 2006 regional company job that I started upon moving to the mid-west; I made a judgment error, perhaps the pregnancy hormones, but I own it. It was me. I was put on a PIP during this regional company tax senior job. I was struggling to keep up technically but at least fulfilling a tax staff level of capacity and always a pleasant team player. These technical issues were getting incrementally better but then I made a major judgment error that was the inflexion point of putting me in a PIP situation fairly quickly. I had looked for sympathy from the HR director when my tax partner boss was too candid with me one afternoon. He had said "Alayna, you wouldn't survive" in reference to the fact I had made some continuous calculation errors with a tight time crunch project and rushed the end of it. I was falling asleep at my desk with this pregnancy, craving more sugar, sleepy always. Unfocused. The decreased work quality and the overly emotional self were starting to show through.

Again, I didn't follow rank and file and went somewhat above the tax partner's head to HR. It was just a casual conversation with the HR director, I told her: "I'm scared. He said I won't survive." And she responded that said she would talk to this partner. Then and there I should have insisted to her to just keep it between us, I was just venting and it wasn't meant to be a solution oriented request. I'm not sure that would have precluded her from going up the chain to him on it though. HR loyalties cannot be relied upon in certain circumstances. I was looking for understanding or pity – I'm not sure which. I had growing anxiety about losing this job. I had needed to touch base with HR given the upcoming disability leave for maternity time and this was a side comment when she asked how everything is going. I should have kept my mouth shut.

People like me with little or no fatherly presence in childhood statistically are said to have trouble with recognizing authority in our adult years. I should have known better though. I needed to be in the US legitimately, and I was still on an H1B visa at this time. My husband had sponsored me, but the application was stuck for years. Jeopardizing my employment by commiserating to the HR director was an overly emotional and miscalculated step.

It became personal for the tax partner after he found out I had talked with the HR director about his comment; it became a vendetta for him to get rid of me. I get that now, but around those years I was spiteful at the thought of him. In retrospect I realize though that he had invested a lot of time developing my tax knowledge and skills. This was a knife in the back to him. I wasn't doing a great job to begin with; the confidence never came. The knowledge was there, but the confidence itself didn't break through. I was a tax senior and the paranoia of failure and judgment was always a dark cloud over me. All the tax knowledge I gained from him was sitting dormant in my head but never translated into actual skills. The tax partner's performance review of me was written in such a horridly mean manner, my husband was shocked as well, at the lead in it when I showed Darrell.

Here I was a second time; both on probation and pregnant. I had tried very hard; I had a publicly traded company's (one listed on the stock exchange) return due June 15th and worked two nights till 3:00 a.m. and was back in the office again at 7:00 a.m. I had to elevate my feet on a box while at my desk working because of painful sciatica. I made it through the meticulous and voluminous tax preparation. A fellow staff lady who had been promoted to manager was in awe of my efforts and mentioned that to me. "Alayna, I admire you for that." She reviewed some of my work, and it was still messy. The software and dealing with IRS Section 179 and bonus depreciation adjustments across thirty-seven state tax returns was killing me compounded with my lack of confidence and overwhelming tiredness from the pregnancy hormones.

The company was good to me in that they kept me on their benefit plan and with disability pay until after my maternity leave that was again just eight weeks. I was expected to depart thereafter and not come back.

I went back to the previous offer out of the convenience of it. I was raising a toddler and infant and doing a deep dive into a large job search was just insurmountably difficult at that time. I instead searched and dug up an email from two years prior where the local three-hundred person CPA firm had emailed me an offer letter for a tax manager position. I replied back to that same string, so it would be instant for them to remember they'd made me an offer. I interviewed within a couple of days while a heaving nine months pregnant to secure a position in winter after maternity leave. It was the only interview in which I didn't wear a business suit. I apologized for being underdressed, and they had chuckled warmheartedly.

I had also scheduled to have Hudson after the extended corporate tax due date in September similar to Madison's timing, so I wouldn't miss any critical tax work that could help demonstrate performance and possibly earn a crucial growth period that would facilitate a future promotion. I really wanted to climb that now very steep corporate ladder. But I slipped at every rung, and maybe was only on rung two at this point 7 years in. Not even that far up maybe.

The new company was a blessing in that it was part time. Flexible time schedule was their claim to fame as a company with local female CPAs. They even had a male in tax who worked part time as he managed his family's business on the side. Flex-time was helpful as Hudson wasn't sleeping through the night until he was five months. I had put him on cereal at eight weeks, like I had done with Maddy. I had asked the nurse about this too, as they say no solid foods till six months. The nurse had said, "Look, we have to tell you for liability reasons, no, not until they have the chewing reflex, but I did it at eight weeks as a mom. You figure out what you need to do." I was thankful for her candid advice. The cereal didn't work to put Hudson to sleep throughout the night though. So it was a situation of downing a lot of coffee to get through the work day.

    Hudson would be up a couple times at night. Two nannies quit on me as Bethany and her husband who both had a language barrier would always be hovering as surveillance over them. These nannies quit and left with no notice each time, just making excuses why they couldn't come in the next day or the day after that. It was stressful having to infringe on getting the parents help as they were already far up in their elder years. Busy season was a situation of me being fueled by caffeine and surviving on broken sleep. I was full time in busy season. Then tapered down outside busy season. By the time I was going into the second busy season, Hudson was one and Madison four. Bethany and her husband were much older now and it was difficult for them to take care of Hudson while I worked but they persevered and stayed with us the first ten months in our large mid-west home.

    In the second January with this firm, I was told by my manager secretively that there was a huge lawsuit at the company brought upon them by a former client, and one-third of the staff will lose their jobs. I was officially at a staff level there since I was part time but operating and categorized as a senior with senior level pay and responsibility. In tandem with this event, my close colleague at work was struggling and about to be let go. It was the same thing as me years ago; they weren't giving her feedback. Looking at her I saw a flashback of me when I was at the Multinational CPA firm and no one told me what I was doing wrong until annual review time. My remorse crept in, but I should have minded my own business.

I was starting to feel manic over losing a job if there were indeed going to be layoffs due to the lawsuit. Meanwhile this work friend of mine had brought up how she was struggling and the managers had given her a really bad review and weren't helpful in the least when she had questions. I made the mistake of going out on a limb and told this fellow lunch buddy, "You probably should look for another job if you feel this one is in jeopardy. It's easier to find something else while still employed." She appreciated that, at least on the surface of it. But then it put her into a sort of resentment frenzy with her superiors over not being thoroughly taught by her immediate supervisors. All of this happened in a blur of a couple of weeks; and I sent an email to my boss, after the layoff speculation was laying heavily on me. I had written to him the back story on what my manager had told me, and that I was not sure why she was telling me this and that it seemed quite negative and created a lot of uncertainty for staff. I sent the email on a Friday and lost sleep all weekend as I received no response and was thus full of anxiety.

On Monday the managing partner and my immediate boss brought me in for questioning. "So your manager said that?" They realized it was bad judgment on the manager's part to say anything about the lawsuit and she was no doubt reprimanded afterwards. Her face went beet red when she later passed my cubical and looked away. After questioning on this lawsuit incident, the managing partner also brought up that I shouldn't have talked to my colleague about finding another job. He said I had gone out on a limb by doing that. He was right.

I had encouraged her to save herself from being unemployed like me in the past, I thought to myself. She was in fact let go a year later. When she raised her concern to the managing partner, he likely cut her some slack, perhaps got her the feedback help she needed. I learned she was unemployed for many months before finding something else. It's likely she had bought some time for herself, complaining to the managing partner about the lack of feedback. You have to make the most of that next honeymoon period they give you though.

    I cried in that meeting with the immediate boss and the managing partner. I was low on sleep and having my manic self try to keep together the household, infant, toddler, forty-minute commute, busy season, and constant sleep deprivation. Keeping up everything like the over-productive American mom's expectation of themselves goes. Bethany and her husband had gone back to India by now to close up their home and wrap up their assets in order to move to America permanently but it was a long process and they couldn't be here with us. I was falling apart. When I can control it I avoid showing strong emotion at work. When you cry at work it's like you lose all your respect and power. I had already lost my grip however and was sobbing audibly in front of two partners in that closed office.

    My husband didn't let me go back to work this time after a month, which was a good thing. We waited four months. We didn't make that mistake again. Although at the time, I wanted to go back after a month. I felt fine, but that judgment wasn't there; I learned this for myself after this episode. Darrell already knew I wasn't fully functional yet in a cognitive way. I had to go through it myself and be aware of it to truly believe it.

    With February arriving, I went on FMLA at that point after the teary breakdown in the partner's office, and my colleagues didn't know what was happening. One of my colleagues had reached out to me, but I never responded. I was too scared. What do I say? I'm having a mental breakdown? A bipolar episode? That would become the talk of a now four-hundred-person firm; they had grown rapidly because of acquisitions of smaller firms.

    This time the component of the company that processed disability payments was in fact the onsite HR department, not an offsite location like the situation had been in the Multinational firm. So my office's HR department had to be told I had bipolar disorder from the doctor's note and was to process the time off and disability pay. The HR director said he absolutely would not tell my bosses after I asked him to please not tell of my diagnosis. He said, "By policy, we don't." They probably figured it out anyways in the core services group, from the erratic and pressured fast speech that had started in those last few days while still at work.

My husband asked me pointedly, "Are you going to believe the HR director? Really? He will definitely tell the bosses." This time he was the wiser for it, the first time I went back after a month of FMLA. This time I was chomping at the bit to go back after one month and help in busy season. But we waited till after April 15th tax deadline. I fought with Darrell. This would look horrible! It would look unacceptable to a team that didn't know what was going on, and it likely enraged them that they had to weather the additional workload of someone last minute without explanation. These things are planned for and staff is hired well before tax season starts. It left them overworked and in a pickle.

The core services group likely thought it was a convenient hiatus from busy season. They likely speculated it was an excuse on my part of feigning a random illness or family emergency so I could just skip the tough tax season and raise my small children comfortably without the busy work hours. It was an invisible thought bubble I pictured in the team's mind that Alayna is getting paid to sit out busy season and then will come back during the downtime season once it is convenient for her. Alayna must be playing some family emergency disability card to not have to share this workload. I'm thinking the worst of what they might have assumed but it likely wasn't anything empathetic.

I was too ashamed to tell the colleague who reached out and expressed concern while I was out on leave – on the reality of what had happened. She was a tenured flex-time superstar at the firm and a fair amount of maturity about her as she raised a large family and worked longer hours in busy season. There were so many stigmas with mental illness at that time though, and there still is today. I had bipolar disorder and if I told her there was no undoing that secret ever. There was no getting that genie back in the bottle. I did yearn to respond to her, but never did. There was nothing I could say that would help the colleagues understand what I was going through without attaching stigma to me forever. In hindsight sometimes I wonder if I had just told her I was having a "stress breakdown" maybe that would have been relatively stigma free. But that term never came to my mind, just the weight of my bipolar label stayed at the top of my mind. My colleagues must have thought I faked an emergency with family. I never responded to her email. I was hoping to become a manager at this firm one day. I could write that off now completely. I was still on that second rung of the corporate ladder.

Likely because of the recent medical leave, the company couldn't terminate me immediately upon arrival back or that would expose them to some legal issues where an employee comes back from disability and is terminated promptly.

Culturally this firm was different than the other firms I'd worked for in the past. There was a level of toxicity in the management ranks as with a manager breaking protocol and telling subordinate level staff about layoffs. The manager shouldn't have been talking to even a senior, or a staff about anything confidential like that. The culture was also different in that, compared to the organic culture of the regional company, it was a boys' club mentality with some sexual innuendo from male partners at the top of the organization. It wasn't the place for me anyways.

I never told Darrell till years later what my immediate partner boss kept asking of me. "Let's go have a bottle of wine" and "We should work out together" had been some of the things coming out of his mouth that I'd brush off. This partner would complain about his wife to me. That was a huge red flag as well – he was on the prowl all the time. I didn't want Darrell to think I was causing this behavior in the partner. I never mentioned it to him while I was there. I've realized men like this partner are simply looking to play. Women whom they shower attention upon should be aware and never think they'll leave their wife for a side relationship. They don't want to split half with an X, and they generally love their kids. Getting sucked into this type of relationship may not yield anything other than disappointment. If the man can betray his wife he can betray another woman too. I see women get snaked into relationships like this, thinking the guy will give her financial security and faithfulness. I have witnessed with these relationships too that they seldom are long lasting companionships but just an enthralling escapade.

This male boss was annoying. He'd call as soon as he saw I was online and ask me to come to his office and to also close the door behind me.

I had done an excellent technical job here with accuracy and interpreting tax law specific to client situations. The water had recessed from my head, and I could do easy work compared to the regional company's client roster and complexity. Coming from a heavy tax group that was boot camp to now a generalist group and also stepping down to a staff title where expectations were lower helped me knock it out of the park. But I was sure the office rumors were rampant. An old white guy with privilege and I'm always in his office with the door closed. It made the whole situation feel cheap on a daily basis.

June came, and there were several waves of layoffs after busy season as the mortgage crisis recession of 2010 hit. My managing partner set a meeting with me about needing to set an end date, as I couldn't find any other employment that they had already suggested I find a month prior. They were pushing this on me due to "client loss." They would never say it was because they are worried about my mental stability. I'm sure it was the latter, someone doing good technical work otherwise isn't let go easily.

By now, luckily I had acquired green card status, as my husband had become a citizen and upgraded his application. After that status change my application rolled forward much quicker. I sent my farewell email to my core services group of people, and after one week wound down and boxed up my belongings for home.

To illustrate the grandiose thoughts of this illness, during Hudson's postpartum period episode, I thought President Obama had installed a special information tower near my home, as I was to be controlling all the Central Intelligence Agency's matters for the government. It was in fact just a new electrical pole. But I truly believed it was for me. The world revolves around you when you have that bipolar manic feeling of grandiosity. I hear things sometimes that are not there which are a symptom of bipolar disorder mania. This hallucination symptom occurs in schizophrenia additionally.

I would be completely delusional in my grandiose self. My Dad was the same way. Sitting in the back of a cop car once, the cops told Mom afterward that Dad had joked he must be the king and they must be his servants driving him to his palace. Grandiosity, it is such a bad virtue, a dangerous one, an embarrassing one. It is one that haunts you with its regrettable and awkward memories for life.

I ask my husband sometimes about his feelings toward having to manage my illness. I feel sorry for him at times. "On a daily basis are you anticipating the next episode?"

He said, "Yes, during those times it's here… It's top of mind. Otherwise outside that it's not a daily concern."

I've been insecure with Darrell every time a job loss has happened and I have no income. I am insecure when that work identity is lost. I feel like he's disgusted with me, and I'm abrasive back. It's all in my head though – but I don't realize that at the time. As long as the house and kids are doing well, he's unconcerned if I work now. He's doing well in his career. We don't need two incomes at this point. Part of him knows me working a high paying high stress job creates more problems than it answers for our family.

My doctor says my medication dosages are on the lower end of an average dosage regimen typically prescribed to those suffering from bipolar disorder. Perhaps my diagnosis was caught early enough in life and treated with lower doses and still effective; perhaps it negated the need for heavier medications and dosages like in my dad's case where he was on very heavy doses. He was diagnosed much later in his life. I'm not sure why the vast difference in mine and his medication strengths other than the age of when the treatment started for each of us.

I couldn't imagine what it's like for a family who has never dealt with bipolar disorder before and trying to manage a loved one from harming themselves, harming other people, or running outside wildly into traffic and putting yourself and any kids at home in danger. Risky behavior is an issue along with heightened sexual pursuits, substance abuse, alcoholism, etc. I can only guess how bad I make things for my loved ones and try to periodically project myself in their shoes when I'm episode free and reflecting back.

Upon losing the large CPA firm job I could finally drop my load after all those years of being chained to my desk with a work visa over my head. I was a green card holder now. But I would have bursts of sudden energy at home. This was pent up creative energy that had to be applied somewhere. One time I was trying to do a business plan for a personal grocery shopper business as it became my fixation and obsession to earn again at a higher rate than just my unemployment income.

I started to get irritable with my husband over a lot of things during that business plan writing time. I had lost weight at home with the kids, changing diapers on the 2nd floor – running up from the first floor many times a day, and other mothering matters. The weight loss was great. I hit my pre-pregnancy weight. I didn't think I'd ever see those numbers on the scale in my lifetime again.

I closed up the plan, though, once I gained the self-awareness of starting to be bitchy. I saw business owners get divorced all the time, because of the external pressures. This isn't for me. I have a great marriage, and my husband is doing well. Leave it, just mind the kids.

The nicotine cravings had come back during this time at home. It is this feeling in your gut that you'll die without a cigarette. But I found a way around it finally ... During this past busy season episode I had started smoking Darrell's cigarettes again while trapped on disability leave. Mom had flown in twice during these months I sat out busy season and she helped manage the house and kids while I regained judgment. After she left, I had lost the job that summer and was home full time where the cravings still continued and I was sometimes leaving the kids alone in the house, an infant and toddler, to go outside and smoke on the side of the house away from any windows where they could see me. Finally, in 2011 I was able to shake off the feeling of craving it entirely. I was sick of my behavior of putting the kids in danger while I smoked, I was utterly disgusted with myself. I made a promise with God to send me collateral damage—I'm still ashamed to this day to say what that is—if I ever smoke again. I have not craved it since. It was like a light switch went off.

 I had dreams the first ten months after making that promise. Dreams where I'd wake up from it scared I had just smoked and it might happen, the thing I most feared. It was enough to work. I can stand in the middle of smokers, and it doesn't faze me. My husband also quit that year after Hudson was born, because he knew I'd keep going back to it if I had his cigarettes lying around. Making a promise to a higher power I believe in worked for me and has since for ten years now. I don't have any cravings or future desire to smoke anymore. When life happens, I know this could become a vice again, so I sealed off alcohol in that same pact so I didn't turn to another vice to alleviate stress.

 I said to myself, Karma will get you if you smoke again. It goes like this, and maybe it will work for someone else out there too. Imagine the worst fear and that it will come true if you smoke again. Make a pact with that higher power you have utmost faith in, and that the higher power will indeed make your fear a reality as you requested of them if you break that promise. As a mother you know what that worst fear is.

 2010 had been a bumpy year, and the only good that came out of it was that Darrell had quit smoking on account of me and hopefully would stay healthy for life. The next year was about to arrive and so was another opportunity for tax busy season work. Since my unemployment insurance payments could be stretched a bit more if I worked temporarily in between as a contract employee I was strongly considering working again. Additionally finding some contract work to show continuity of working busy seasons on my resume would help. I also thought potentially a company I could join for busy season would offer me a full-time job afterwards too if I was good.

I applied to a busy season posting at a multi-state CPA firm with offices in neighboring states, and this company's local office was about a half hour away from home. They never offered me a full-time job, and I don't think I asked them either. They had enough people to keep busy when work was sparse and sporadic for tax professionals in the off season; so it helped to offload my seasonal payroll burden after tax season ended. Thus I wasn't offered a job although I was exceeding expectations by delivering accurate project work and it was always under time budget which helped the company's margins. The no job offer was a blessing in disguise as my children were missing their mom direly.

Bethany and her husband came from the West Coast during this busy tax season. By this time they had sold everything overseas and moved to the US; it wasn't safe for an older couple like them to live alone in India, their kids felt. They were here to take care of Maddy and Hudson, as I worked fifty hours a week in that tax season. I no longer did the sixty- to eighty-hour work weeks like when I had been tethered to a work visa and could only stick to full time jobs that would hire me based on a cumbersome expensive visa application an employer would have to compile. I had the safety net of a husband and a green card now. This busy season job was a break away from baby world that I had been in for six months now. But the childcare wasn't easy for Bethany, who ended up doing everything around the house. I was gone Saturdays too. On Sunday I didn't even want to look at housework or cooking. She was so sweet that way and had a lot of energy to continue to handle things at home. But it wore on her too. She was developing rheumatoid arthritis during those years.

Having an active CPA license I felt propelled me to work busy season. The unemployment income capped out at only $363 weekly – that was the maximum one can get. With the CPA license I felt I couldn't just sit at home; I was meant for more than just child diapering. Those insecure thoughts would start to creep in as the months went by.

Around these years where I bounced busy season jobs; we realized my Dad had vascular dementia. Dad's history had a sad irony even before this diagnosis. Years ago he was living in a retired veteran's assisted living apartment building in downtown Vancouver where they served meals and had a cleaning lady come in. However it had cockroaches in places and money went missing from my dad's room all the time. My husband and I went to visit him in 2015 and this time at his residence. Dad's apartment, which consisted of only one single room and a bathroom, was in the bad part of downtown. He had always visited everyone in another part of town but when Darrell and I went we told him we would come to him.

Dad was starting to forget when Delilah would call him to come down to the SkyTrain stop in her part of town to visit the grandkids, like he usually did every so often. His part of town was too dangerous. She'd never been there with her four little kids. But I visited there in 2015 for the first time, and that's when my older sister and I figured we had to move him out of there as soon as possible. Delilah moved Dad to her suburb, to an assisted living apartment, with its own living space apartment units on higher floors and a joint eatery on the main floor. It was clean and luxurious looking. It looked like the Conrad hotel compared to where he was before.

Dad would spill his tea on the wall behind the garbage bin as he discarded the tea bag into the kitchen trash. There was always a lot of mess to clean up for Delilah. Emilia was still in Alberta.

It was all up to Delilah to maintain Dad's place. She somehow managed to run two households for half a year with four kids, two of which were infant and toddler age.

We didn't know at that point that Dad had vascular dementia, until the police picked him up one day when he was taking his usual walk outside in the tree-lined suburb and became lost. He couldn't find his way back. A couple times prior to this, strangers would pick him up in their car—it was a nice part of town—and bring him to his apartment complex. But when the police noticed his confusion and had to help him get home, they instead took him to the hospital. It was the same hospital where two decades earlier I had been admitted twice to its psychiatric ward.

An MRI was done, and it was found that Dad had had multiple mini-strokes over the years, and the oxygen wasn't getting to his brain properly. It was something about brain blood vessels thinning out because of these multiple small strokes. That's when the provincial government moved him from hospital to nursing home.

My Dad still says to this day he wants to be reunited with his mother and die at age 63, the same age that his mother was when she died. He's made it over a decade beyond that. His vascular dementia and wandering has meant his confining to this nursing home's lockdown side for the past many years. He is forgetting most of the people in his life and what he did two hours ago. Nursing homes aren't typical for subcontinent elders. But Dad was a violent man for decades. No one could be expected to take that risk into their home and put their own family into danger. He once ran after my mom with a knife. I can't wipe that memory from the mining town days. She hid behind a mahogany-colored door, trying to save herself by putting pressure on it with her weight; there was no lock.

His nursing home entrance meant his meals were carefully measured, medicines were on time, bathing was regular and dental hygiene was monitored. His lifestyle was far from healthy prior to that. While downtown for decades, he had a habit of eating once a day, a large buffet meal, maybe to save money, I think. Even when at the veteran's apartment, which was open to all geriatric men, he didn't eat their prepared food. He'd go to an Indian buffet in the same part of town instead. He had run up quite a tab at the Indian restaurant also. When Mom finally was able to sell the Vancouver home and Dad received his $100,000 portion from it —only that much because they deducted the child support he never paid—his younger brother had to settle his huge tab with the Indian country men who owned that particular buffet downtown.

Dad walked a good deal in the worst part of town, the Hastings Street area of Vancouver, where the local rumor was that AIDS started there in the 1970s. Dad liked it there though. He could handle when trouble walked his way, he had told me his strategy was to put forth a pack of cigarettes and say to the thug, "Hey, man, have a cigarette," and smile warmly. That would instantly de-arm any of their possible bad intentions and turn these men or women friendly.

They would say to him, "Thanks, what's your name? You need anything, bro, you let me know." And he would often be later solicited by them to buy stolen goods. He always wanted to stay in the bad part of town although the government would have paid his rent the same way in a better part of town. We'd always encourage him to move to a better part of town but he said he felt like he belonged there amongst those kinds of people. I think deep down he felt he was still a winner amongst the most downtrodden of the local human race and perhaps it gave him a self of normalcy and confidence.

Dad managed his medications himself, and when his mom died in early 2003, he was severely episodic again. Dad's younger brother, Zachary, who was immediately younger than him in the line of six siblings, would always come to his rescue and have his pills organized in a bagged kit, following him closely. Uncle Zachary loved Dad so much, and I realized he'd always wanted his older brother's approval – perhaps that's why Uncle Zachary would weather Dad's insults to him and show him undue compassion even with Dad's constant unmasked animosity towards him.

My Dad always spat anger unfairly at Uncle Zachary; this was out of jealousy and insecurity. Uncle Zachary had done well for himself. He had built expansive real estate over the years. He also owned multiple taxi cabs and their licenses from the best taxi cab company in greater Vancouver. He was well off for over twenty years now since the 1990s, all in an admirably blue collar way. This was before Uber. I heard each cab license was worth over a hundred thousand dollars to own the rights to drive for the prestigious cab company that serviced mainly downtown and airport clientele. I was told that amount – I didn't corroborate the value. The Indian community has a habit of exaggerating by quite a multiple factor. Regardless though, it was still a lot of wealth Uncle Zachary had accumulated, and he had done well for himself. He had done so with no college education but a lot of grit, hard work and long hours.

Uncle Zachary always had shown Dad a lot of affection and care, often going to the nursing home and taking him out for a shave and hair cut routinely. It's a mystery if any of his other siblings ever visited Dad. In addition to his siblings he had thirty-plus nieces and nephews in the Vancouver area. But life gets busy and it is not their prerogative to visit him but I hope they do on occasion. Since he has a short memory of two hours, he can't tell me whether anyone has come by or not. He's alone most days, looking out his window into the parking lot and trees lining it. But he says he's happy there. Sadly he has been forgotten by most of the rest of his family other than Uncle Zachary. He has been forgotten by those other four siblings who he had helped settle and bring to the new world. He was an integral part of making their lives better. I earnestly hope they do visit him at times even out of empathy.

I sometimes discuss with Delilah whether we made the right decision to put him in the nursing home where he was assigned to the lock down side for those patients who could wander away and not come back. His admittance there is for his safety and longevity, but we worry it's become a mundane existence and there is definitely a significant trade-off in the lifestyle of a nursing facility contrasted with his free roaming days when he enjoyed going wherever he liked along the downtown skyline, parks and seawall. Agreed he started needing assistance finding his way back home. That was the main catalyst in the decision to put him where he is now. His life would likely have been shorter roaming free without any managed meal plans and medicinal regimen. But perhaps his life would be more enriched had he stayed out of the nursing care facility. I wonder what Dad would have chosen for himself had he been in a decision making capacity. There are a plethora of mixed feelings Delilah and I have about Dad staying in the care facility and his only pass time being looking out the window to the trees lining the parking lot. He does not participate in any of the nursing home's activities or engage with the other individuals who mostly appear far past the stage of coherence, unlike him – an inpatient that can still rattle off rhyming couplets and engage in active and timely conversation.

Dad had hit me only twice in my life, the second time being during Grandma Edna's funeral. I hadn't yet elaborated on the first time though; it had been when I was age four. I was entirely asking for it in that particular instance. I had literally hugged to death two snow-white baby bunny rabbits he had bought for me and Delilah. One died in the car while we were bringing it home from the farm that sold them. Delilah and I were turned around facing the hatchback's trunk without seatbelts on and we were leaned over the backseat playing with the bunnies and I specifically was starting to hug them in a hyper manner. The remaining rabbit died while my dad was making a cage for the surviving one down in the garage. My mom went down and said solemnly, "Paul, you can stop now; there's no point. Alayna's killed the second one too." Dad was in a rage when he came upstairs and gave me a small smack. Years later he would bring up the smack multiple times while tearful and say he regretted hitting me on such an unimportant matter. He was tormented by it and would tell me: "They were just some damn bunnies."

I wonder now, was there some aggression tied to bipolar predisposition that led me as a child to kill these animals while playing with them or just an honest mistake in the moment's excitement? I hope it was the latter.

I recall what might be another tinge of slight bipolar symptoms in me as a child. I had a field trip in grade three to Dad's mineral mine, and I cried when I didn't see my dad, cried on the two hour bus ride all the way home. He had indeed waved at me, I was told later. I did that as a kid, cried a lot when I was alone, this mining incident was tangible and perhaps the crying was understandable but I was obsessively fixated on the self pity of it; besides this disproportionately emotional instance there were other times where for no apparent reason my thoughts would make me sad. The sadness wasn't revolving around a particular event though, it was just one thought leading to the next and something sad felt consistently along the way. I felt alone in the world but at the same time the world was only meant for me, I was the center of it and only God was focused on me, and no one else. That recurrent thought I recall even now – it's a thought that would follow me during long car rides and road trips. I remember the tears that would come especially on these longer car rides where I would be looking away from everyone out the window. Maybe this was an indication of bipolar disorder, when one is sad without a reason to be sad, coupled with the grandiose feeling that the world was revolving around me solely and only existed for me. I was a stubborn, headstrong kid with disobedience and oppositional behavior. It was markedly difficult for my mom to manage my behavior along with all the other stressors in her life so I'd be spanked a lot. Then there was this short lived depression of sorts in the car when nothing really had happened to cause tears to roll down but just the thoughts in my head were enough to push me into a silent crying frenzy. I speculate whether that was an early sign of something not right with me.

Decades later these qualities I watched for like a hawk in my own kids and my husband would keep dissuading me from it. "You are over-diagnosing," he'd say.

Clinically one of my psychiatrists said it is normal for a bipolar patient to hit an episode in the first year after delivery of a child; and that's exactly what happened. I had two episodes in those post pregnancy years, and roughly at the nine-month and one-and-a-half-year marker. I wish I had diagnosed the onset of those situations better.

The postpartum time after bearing an infant is definitely a precarious one for a worker during a busy time like tax season, compounded with responsibilities of managing a household, daycare, and eighty-hour work weeks. Add to these factors the additional burden of bipolar disorder. A long hiatus from work may have been very beneficial in order to keep stable and preserve an untainted impression amongst my employer in lieu of just an eight week leave after having a child.

Chapter 13

Fraud Anxiety

2011

My ninth job was at a small local firm that offered both accounting and attorney services. This firm was sued by a former client for a sales tax liability oversight. One of the men in charge of the practice was asked to leave. He had worked on the file associated with the oversight that caused the client millions of dollars in a missed tax liability. He had to be terminated by the owner of the firm who was both a CPA and attorney. Otherwise if this man stayed with the firm, the professional liability insurance company would skyrocket the premiums beyond affordability. The man at fault, then second in command, was asked to find another job, and in two months he found an excellent one and moved to another city.

I was asked to take his place but was very intimidated by the prospect. I struggled to fill his shoes, and there were no other options for a colleague to step up in house. At the part-time, local giant CPA firm, I had excelled as the water had recessed, and I had my head above it finally. However here the work was different; it was an added job description of what I hadn't done before; back office HR, live payrolls, cash management, managing multiple staff, high volume billing and invoicing review, and the list went on.

The CPA/Attorney owner was exhausted with the departure of his second in command and my nervous incompetence. He didn't have the bandwidth to handhold me; he told me in so many words two months in my new role. I suffered with low confidence in trying to run tasks and functions I had never managed solely before with no mentoring assistance. The alpha I assisted made it look so easy earlier.

    I was more of a tax thinker, black and white. I was suddenly managing clerks and bookkeepers and making buying decisions for high-net-worth people and tracking their plane charges based on mileage to see if the shared private jet had charged the right fees, etc.

    The owner had to get someone in there, and fast. A young fellow who had a family to feed and was the sole breadwinner at home was brought in. He carefully reviewed the client lists and their financial details before accepting, as he was going to inherit the accounting side, and the owner was going to continue with just the legal side as he was approaching retirement.

    The young man had me sign the new offer letter paperwork, so I was now under his company. The main purpose for having a new agreement was to have a non-compete and no solicitation agreement in place. There wasn't one done previously when I first started with the firm. He gleaned information on the clients from me that next busy season, and that following summer he fired me. I was choked to overhear this young man talking to someone on the phone, "She's just here to collect a paycheck." He thought I'd left for the evening, and his door was open. I was saddened as I was already working seventy hours weekly. My kids missed me, but this wasn't part time. I was getting paid more than I'd ever made before. And they'd increased me from $65,000 to $75,000 when the alpha guy had left who was making $100,000. The attorney owner didn't want me leaving either, as the young man hadn't come on yet, and he had not found a successor so far that could quarterback the accounting side fully. He didn't want me to depart, at least not yet. As a knee jerk reaction the owner gave me the pay raise as enticement and also in desperation that I would stay on. When I started struggling, he put the feelers out to sell that accounting side of the practice – he had previously offered it to me but I had said no, I didn't want to be a business owner and worry about other people's payroll. I knew I wasn't cut from that cloth.

The pay increase was the owner's insurance for me to stay. And now I became this young man's problem. He was a coward. He didn't even bring me into his office during termination. While I was out for the day because of Maddy and Hudson's doctor office appointments I just received an email from him that I had been terminated. Additionally he had typed that I could pick up my personal belongings at the front desk at some point, and also that my access had been terminated from all systems.

This young man was uncomfortable with firing anyone. He had been a previous regional CPA firm manager and was good at what he did. However HR issues are a scary beast to deal with and they take another kind of grit to terminate someone face-to-face. That would have been new to him. In the bigger firms, the heavies do that. Managers just report the information up the pole. They are typically never sitting in on those final termination meetings – usually that's the HR director and a very senior level person like a partner. So an email was all I got – not the courtesy of a final meeting. It would have been too weird and outside his comfort zone for him.

Darrell took us to Disney World a couple months later, that October. I'd lost my job in early August. My parents had always wanted to take us to Disney, but on a miner's wage it was too expensive to fly from the north western part of Canada, to Florida's Disney World. Even though Dad had good paychecks as he would always take the overtime shifts that paid time and a half when others would call in sick. But he would spend a lot too, in typical bipolar spending-spree style. Money was spent on wasteful items, like excessive lotto tickets, furniture, or tables he liked on a whim. My mom was frustrated. Home was not a warehouse to be overly stuffed with a mish-mash of unnecessary goods and furniture. Mom also felt lotto tickets were an utter waste, a pipe dream of becoming an overnight millionaire.

Finally, in my mid-thirties I was able to experience Disney World. I was able to live its joy vicariously through my children. I had always wanted to take my mom there after visiting and experiencing it, but she can't walk very well given her severe knee problems at her age now. It saddens me that Mom never was able to see it in her life so far, and she's in her mid-sixties now.

Darrell, Maddy, Hudson, and I also went to Universal Studios. I had read all seven *Harry Potter* books—and that theme park was meaningful and amazing to me. I told the rest of my family about each object, building, and character. Darrell isn't much of a reader, especially not fiction. So he just smiled and nodded, but I'm sure he was half-listening but happy at my healthy excitement.

After Disney World, that winter, I found an amazing work-from-home accounting company headquartered on the West Coast. I can still remember that work-from-home accounting company vividly, I was very fond of the people and processes there. I was there for five years and perhaps getting complacent near the end as my clients were very easy and in rhythm, and I was bored and asked for more work. Indeed ask and you shall receive; they gave me the complexity I wanted but that I was not groomed for. What I miss about that company most is the sisterhood camaraderie amongst the controllers and senior controllers, all women in their forties and fifties. I was the baby of the group, joining them at age thirty-four. It felt like home. I was also working from home, an added bonus of a commute that was just a flight of steps to the home office.

I was at this job for a longer duration, five years, before being let go. This was a job I was positive I was going to retire from. But in my fifth year, I got fired again. I refused to continue on a client account that a previous controller had also stepped down from, as she felt the owner of the company's books we managed was unethical. There was some overly optimistic reporting to investors of financials that wasn't the true picture. There were liabilities that were missing. The company hadn't paid its payroll trust liabilities—the employee's withholdings of their federal and state taxes—to the Internal Revenue Service (IRS) in years. They had engaged a settlement company to negotiate with the IRS for a payment plan to buy them some time, but the owner had said he'd close that company during the year so he wouldn't be on the hook for the employer portion. You are bonded personally as an owner to pay the employee portion. But the employer portion could be walked away from if the company was closed I was told. My staff on the account kept looking at me and asking why we were even doing his books. It just felt wrong. But he was doing what a lot of companies do, apparently, to have IRS taxes written off – the owner of my virtual accounting company told me as such. Some of this tax law was above my head, but it didn't feel right. My bosses were okay with it though, however I was at the shaky helm of sending the financials each period.

 I lost a weekend's sleep over needing to send investors' financials on Monday. I sent an email to the directors, saying I can't do it, I want to be removed, and here's my reasons. I was told by the director, "No, you'll have to stay on it, and I can be the heavy on the phone calls with the client if it helps." Employees were asking for pay stubs that this owner didn't have. He was giving them net paychecks and never paying the taxes. It was stressful being on this account. The director said, "It already moved from Cindy over to you. We can't keep moving it." The fees for this client were a few thousand dollars for monthly fractional accounting services of a bookkeeper and controller. The accounting company didn't want to lose the client.

 I called the American Institute of Certified Public Accountants (AICPA) ethics line anonymously a couple weeks later for a second opinion after talking with Cindy, the fellow controller who had the account previously. Cindy was a Generally Accepted Accounting Principles (GAAP) heavyweight controller with thirty years behind her. She had stepped off the account previously, and I had consulted with her about the fishiness before I had raised the issue with my director and as a last resort called the anonymous ethnics hotline at the AICPA as an additional sounding board. During our phone call, Cindy referenced the AICPA slides from a prior year ethics webinar, which said if you know as a CPA it's not right that you should be handling the account and keeping it, document you're advising against such treatments to the client and let the client go. She had said that's why she had stepped down from it. For Cindy it was a phone conversation with the owners and director that she didn't want to handle the client anymore. They had obliged her. I was pigeon-holed with being the second controller wanting off of it and the director I reported to just wasn't getting my discomfort over it. So I put my concerns in an email. I know the director would run circles around me during a live call and convince me to keep it if I had just had a phone call with him instead of an email exchange. He had a tendency to do that with staff – twist it back the other way to be sure his way stands. My stance was an email seemed safest and most convincing to make my case.

    I felt like the company didn't value me as Cindy had asked to step down from it, and they honored her request, but then gave it to me and made me stay on it, ignoring my appeals. I was looking for additional work when I took a client I knew nothing about. Everything else in my revenue book was taking me very little time now, even with a revenue book of over sixty five clients and twenty seven bookkeepers to manage, twelve of which were direct reports. But in my emotions, I felt the company valued Cindy's wishes and not mine. I must be disposable to them. But what I should have kept top of mind were some words of wisdom a friend of mine told me years prior, to remember that a company owes you nothing and you owe the company nothing. There is no guaranteed loyalty either way. If they don't like you, you're out. If you don't like them, you leave.

    When I called the AICPA, I didn't give any names of companies. The expert at the ethics hotline after hearing the fact pattern had said the company was aiding and abetting, and my only avenue was to leave the company to get out of the situation. We get these calls all the time he said, and it's not easy for the CPA, but at that point, there's only that option. It's like client-lawyer privilege but client-CPA privilege. Confidentiality is maintained. But move on.

Yes, there are circumstances where one must report to the authorities or whistle blow; it's an uphill battle, not for a person that has bipolar disorder. It's a storm to weather for years. Anxiety and stress that would feed into mania and a breakdown of family life yet again. Suicides happen; harm happens. A world of paper and money can have its catastrophic effects on flesh and blood that is alive. My yardstick is different on what I can weather. It's not a battle worth fighting.

I often reflect that I'm glad I didn't go into the medical world. The stakes are too high—an operation that goes wrong, a needle not given with a steady hand but instead a shaky one that is manically sleep deprived. That's why CPAs are paid less; no one loses an arm if a filing is missed. You're out some money and penalties, that's all. I can sleep better at night in this profession, at least most nights…

When I emailed about my step down from the fraudster client, my direct boss, the director, got a bee up his bonnet about me immediately. It quickly became a witch hunt. I had great reviews every year for each of the four years prior. For the first time in my career, I had reviews that were meeting and in some areas exceeding expectations.

But suddenly I became his investigation as I had put in writing I would not send the financials via email. That became company liability, if ever there was an issue where investors questioned and lost money from this client's company – there was an email warning in writing about this matter that the company had chose to ignore. This hadn't just been a verbal step down; there was a paper trail in which your staff said they wouldn't do something as it didn't seem right to them. Investors could have sued the firm later if they lost money in this venture. They were basing their assumptions of profitability based on books that had huge holes in them and I was not allowed to put notes in the email to investors disclosing the missing pieces either.

The email on stepping down for various reasons on this client inflamed the director and the owners. They had discussed liability exposure amongst them and figured they were in the right, and there was nothing unethical. After all, companies by law can close themselves up and evade the employer portion of taxes anyways, I was told this by the owner of the accounting firm. In this case the client company was north of eight million in overdue taxes. It still seemed like a backdoor way to evade a boatload of taxes and having knowledge of that and allowing it to go past without a wink was beyond my comfort level.

The owners and the director couldn't let me go right away. Since I had cited the fraud reason for a step down on this client – a firing could be seen as retaliation and wrongful dismissal. So I was under file review, each of the sixty five files. I had an annual revenue book of $990,000 amongst my clients that I'd grown over the years. My clients kept referring new companies in their portfolio to me, and clients had friends who had companies that they referred over to our company, as we were doing a stellar job. The bookkeeper did much of the non-complex transactional heavy lifting; I always gave them the kudos during staff meetings. I was there as a support for them. I would review the financials, reconciliations, sales tax, book yearly tax adjustments, and hold client meetings. My clients loved that I was always great on the phone with them and reached out frequently with a personal touch. If a bookkeeper switched off an account as would happen with staffing turnover often or internal department transfers, I was the constant for the clients and they valued that glue. I always made the client feel like I was there and they were taken care of if there were any concerns. If they lost a load of cargo and had a huge loss, I'd call them just to say, "Hey, so sorry. What's your replacement plan and insurance coverage?" Always I'd give them those touch points. In virtual accounting world, you don't want to make the mistake of it feeling like a faceless call center with a giant phone tree, where work is just being processed and only emails ever go back and forth. I felt I also had contributed significantly in maintaining a solid revenue book of long standing clients for even those accounts affected by constant bookkeeper churn.

The director and owners vendetta was to document anything they could find even cosmetically wrong with my files. Recall I had stellar reviews up until year five and suddenly everything became questionable to them. This director who was my immediate boss was documenting me for a misplaced word in the subject line of an email. He was building a file review of trivial matters and cosmetic mistakes. Bringing the mistakes to my attention during periodic calls where the HR director was also present.

If you ever look with a fresh set of eyes, even at the sharpest CPA books, you'll find something that can be adjusted slightly more so. This accounting director was turning over every rock. I will admit I had two recent clients who were above my pay grade (the complex new ones I'd put my hand up and asked for myself) and these were more at the senior controller level of full accrual accounting. The director had known of my struggles with them previously and they were already flagged by him to move to someone that is more of a heavyweight in particular areas when their schedule allows. I had a more tax and modified accrual basis background, not so much full accrual and I had been hired with the understanding to work on high volume low depth client load and mainly cash basis type files. But now this fact had been conveniently forgotten by the director, and those full accrual complex clients I had struggled with and had raised issues on proactively in earlier weeks to this director ironically now I was now under fire for. He had well known these clients were problematic since their on-boarding and had planned to re-house them.

I had done the right thing I felt to ask for more work as I had additional bandwidth after my book of clients was fairly situated and taking me less time, when I got slated to take more complexity the wheels started coming off and I proactively brought that to my director's attention. Suddenly this became fair game to document the issues as well with these more complex clients. You can do depth or volume in accounting but not both. I already had volume, I didn't have much depth on each client, these new complex ones required a deep dive and a skill set I hadn't honed on revenue recognition and what that meant for various clients accounting. My client base was mainly a cash basis set of books. The director knew this, but given the current circumstances of the company owners wanting to get rid of me all this was rolled into those documentation discussions very conveniently. It was unfair and sad. My pay grade was that of an accounting manager and not that of the full accrual senior controllers. There was an extraordinary pay gap; I was hired to manage volume, not complexity. They started judging me to a much higher standard suddenly where I should have been able to shoulder the new complexity without the guidance I kept asking for.

    I'd made mistakes on these more complex clients, and I had sought help from some of the senior controllers earlier in the year as well, but everyone was so busy and had their own giant client base. I had brought it to the director's attention but the director was never able to get to it other than a quick update check-in on the situation currently which didn't help the accounting issues at hand. The owner's philosophy was an overly simplistic one for the management group "Well, you all have a CPA." So there was little empathy for if you still needed to learn something and didn't know it, there was no ownership on the director's part to teach it either. Most of us kept our mouths shut. The CPA profession is similar to other professions in that there are sub-specialties. In the accounting field these can look like tax, finance, audit, etc. and you can not be a master of all.

    All areas I'd questioned and needed help with were documented on the complex clients as my oversights. Beyond these two problem clients out of the sixty five in my book of business, there were the trivial matters like a missing month notation in the line on an email – one email in thousands that go out during the month on my high client volume. For two months I lost weight and was silently persevering and proud of myself that I didn't land myself into an episode. The witch hunt continued and I stayed positive but very strained and continued to be a support to the bookkeepers and service my clients the best I could. However it was a constant battle to stay stable.

On my son's birthday, I got an instant message at 10:00 a.m. in my home office—to join a call with the director. When I arrived on the virtual video conference call, the HR lady was there with him. They couldn't have fired me right after I sent the dissent email a couple months prior; they had to wait a couple months at least so it didn't look like wrongful dismissal stemming from retaliation. The accounting director went through my mistakes that I was typing vigorously on my side screen for my own betterment later. I loved the company and wanted to stay, just not with this client. I asked this director on that video meeting, "Can we consider a PIP so I can work on these areas?" Although I knew a PIP was an excessive measure for the issues brought up.

The director had said, "No, the company feels it best we should part ways."

I swallowed hard, and the top of mind thought for me was that this was a witch hunt, but I never translated verbally to the director or HR lady my feeling although I was chocked and wanted to scream it. I then typed a farewell message to the controller thread online that I was no longer with the firm and had been terminated. The ladies had set up a video conference immediately to absorb the shock; despite two of them the rest of the group had no idea the investigation that had been going on for two months now.

I told them what had been going on for months now, and tearfully I told them as well that I would miss them. This had been the first time I'd found a job where I felt like I belonged. Cindy and my closest colleague who was at my same cash basis accounting level in the controller cohort, Jamaica, had already known for months I was under investigation and horrified their own files might be looked at. What would the director find in theirs if he ever looked?

Jamaica and I had attained a high level of trust between each other over the years, she had often told me she was looking for another job while employed there. We were strangely connected in a way where you usually can't typically build that trust factor with a colleague. Jamaica had asked the director pointedly in a subsequent call with the other controllers that she would want to be a reference for me even though it was outside company policy and the director obliged to it. Shortly after my dismissal Jamaica left the company as she had been planning for a while. Jamaica was a cancer survivor and her perspective on life was amazingly acute, with unflawed prioritization of what truly mattered, and she had sound advice always.

HR emailed all staff immediately about the departure. This is protocol for any voluntary or non-voluntary termination for the company. For virtual security reasons, everyone is notified of a termination. But HR emailed that I'd resigned for personal reasons. I saw that email come in before access was terminated. The HR lady had told me she'd word it that way, but I'd still get severance pay. They knew inside their minds it would cause too much of a ripple in this firm of now hundreds of people, that a committed, high-profile, and seemingly high-performing and newly promoted controller was suddenly fired. So it was covered up as a resignation on my end.

A couple times I had led the whole company meeting as a facilitator. It was like the *Today* show; I made it fun. The owner who never gives kudos emailed me later. He had been hovering in the backdrop on one of the conference calls and was not on camera – I didn't know he was there. "You did a great job." I could light up a room and make people laugh with tasteful well timed humor. Introducing the next speaker with lively transitions; basically master of ceremonies was my thing I found. They had to tell staff I'd resigned. I had numerous texts, email messages, and an actual call from one staff member. Good luck! Is everything okay? How is your family?

A particular staff member direct called my phone two hours before my severance paperwork came in. Later I saw in the severance letter that I wasn't supposed to tell anyone. I had a teary breakdown with this staff member, that I actually got let go. I was close with her to the limited degree you can be with an accountant as a controller. Her son was going through anxiety at school. I would text her anxiety pamphlets they would distribute at my children's school. She and I really looked out for each other with clients and to a personal degree with knowledge sharing on parenting tips. I gave her honest and candid real time feedback professionally. I was a bit paranoid later about telling her what I had told her during those first two hours of being let go. This because once I had the severance contract in hand, I read it through and thought, oh-no, if I want the money, I shouldn't have talked about the termination with a staff person especially more junior than me. But the offer letter was email time stamped 3:43 p.m. I recall vividly, and the accountant had called me at 1:21 p.m. per my iPhone history. If it ever came up, I'd have the evidence ready that I didn't know I was not to say anything at the time of the call as I had not received any paperwork to require as such.

My sixth episode in life was a month after I was let go from this five year job, and this time ironically not *during* the job but in the aftermath. The first three weeks being a SAHM was fun and liberating, and I was relieved not to be the victim of the witch hunt anymore that had lasted two whole months. But then by week four, I realized I was jobless and defunct yet again, holding an active CPA license with nothing professional to work on. My kids were in school during the day. I had nothing to do most of the day after preparing evening dinner and I had not let go of the cleaners. There was not much to do other than dishes, floor cleaning, and waiting for the kids to come home. I didn't like watching TV. An empty mind became a devil's den. My self-worth started depreciating in my mind.

My husband was finding my moods difficult and withdrew, too. He was trying to reduce how much he smoked as he had started again, and I had tallied up his usage from credit card lists and was worried he was hooked again. He was over the threshold of the 15 cigarettes a day that becomes lethal long term. He had quit when I kept going for his cigarettes years prior. But things were stressful again, and he had started back up these past few months. Perhaps he was worried I would be pushed into another episode because of the work situation. He understood my concern for his health and that I didn't want to be widowed early. I needed him. So he was going through his own quiet withdrawal of reducing the habit. He controlled it well, never angry – but just really quiet and sometimes slightly snippety. He just liked the buzz the cigarette gave him especially after a meal. And I understood it was an escape for men – vices like drinking and smoking. Sometimes they can't confide their fears in anyone. Kids have their mom or dad to talk to, women commiserate with one another freely or with their spouses, but men are more often than not solitary creatures who keep their feelings in and don't cry. Although they should, they want to, but societal expectation pressures them against it. So if you can't worry your wife with it, then you lose yourself with the buzz of a cigarette or with the booziness of a bottle.

    Darrell shared a lot with me, but I weaken at times, and he knows when I'm not in my element I can't take any further stresses. Now it was troubling him again; he and I thought I'd keep this job until I retire. His hopes for me on that stability shattered as well, and I wasn't taking being a stay at home mom gracefully either. I was starting to get insecure and overtly mean trying to compensate for my insecurity. The pressure of a sole breadwinner for him came on. Some men typically don't have a problem with being a sole breadwinner. It's the additional pressure of what if something happens to them—what will become of the family—that eats at them more so. I must continue to work and grow enough assets that my family will be okay if I am no longer here.

Darrell had the stress of whether his wife could ever hold down a job and whether he could count on that income for major purchases and retirement funding decisions. He knew he had to do it on his own and leave me at zero dollars on his spreadsheet for planning household income and a thirty-year outlook where he'd figure out the home's early payoff, kids' college, how much to put in retirement each year, etc. He knew my income was just gravy on top but didn't count on it beyond unemployment income level or just zero.

At this stage Darrell wanted me to just be happy. Work or don't work; it's okay… on some level he realized steady secure work historically had always been a challenge for me; to hold any job down seemed unlikely now. He had also believed I would retire at this last job and be able to keep it until I myself chose to leave it. He finally had resolved to understand that I was unreliable for an income source after 15 years and if I was minding the home and kids that would be enough help for him. But I became unsettled with no professional work to do.

People with bipolar disorder take it out on their spouses or their closest loved ones. A mom, a sibling, whoever is trying to care for you the most. It's not easy being the partner of a bipolar person. During this fourth week after losing my job I felt Darrell was being mean to me. I had brought a thermos full of hot chai to an Indian community picnic he was joining after work. I brought the kids. I had asked him if he wanted a cup, and he glared, looked away, and said "no." I was shocked. I thought he was disgusted with me for losing my job. It took a year to realize, no, he was just going through a bit of his own withdrawal of nicotine. Or maybe he had had a bad day at work and didn't feel like conversing, Then there was the time I was disheartened and angry at him for leaving a dry cleaning tag in the walk in closet for days on the carpet as though it was beneath him to pick up his own trash (it was on his side of the closet) and I figured he had left it for me intentionally. I felt demeaned.

On a few trivial things like this and my own compounding feeling of insecurities that were making a monster in my mind about Darrell allegedly mistreating me, I finally flew off the handle with him. I did the silent treatment thing, and it was killing me, but this time I'd keep it going a long time. I was angry – and so insecure and mad. I complained to a friend who was always at odds with her husband, and she gave me well-meaning advice but one that didn't fit my situation. She'd kept her own finances separate and made sure she was in control and suggested I do the same. She lied to her husband a lot too, about where she was in town. She had invited me to a nightclub with another girlfriend that week but had told her husband her best friend was sick and she was with her instead. I recoiled a bit from her during that discussion where she had professed the lies she'd told her husband. That was earlier in the week.

By the end of the week, I slept in a separate bedroom from Darrell. And I was in bad shape but hiding it. I'd stopped sleeping. Coincidently I was out of most of my sleep medicines. Later in life, I had five different sleep medicines—three prescription and two over the counter. But at this juncture I wasn't aware of all the other sedatives out there I could take in combination. Insomnia for a bipolar mind is a freight train that only a sedation injection in the hospital will stop immediately, or the right mixture of strong oral sedatives. An injection is only given in a hospital in the US where heart rate and everything can be monitored; a psychiatric nurse told Darrell that fact once when he had asked about the procedure. So I have to resort to medicines even in an emergency, or I'll pay my entire high deductible from my health plan of $3,500 out of pocket to the hospital even with insurance if I were to go in for such an injection. Insomnia is my hallmark symptom—no sleep for three days—and the gloves come off, in my psychiatrist's words. "You're full manic, Alayna, if you haven't slept the third night. It will take months to regain your balance completely from that."

The silent treatment and its resulting anxiety were starting to feed into my insomnia. The silence I was continuing to give was wearing on me just as much as Darrell. The silence was affecting my sleep. For Darrell the negative effect was he started verbally ripping into the kids about every little reprimand he could find during that week. I missed Darrell, but I wasn't going to be the first to make up. I, myself, resolved that we might have a separation under the same roof till the kids are older, then I'd leave him and be free and travel with girlfriends or find another companion that respected and cared for me and wasn't domineering and rude like a typical Indian man to his wife. These were some extreme thoughts I'd never had before in our milder spats predating this conflict. But Darrell did care. It was my manic mind creating thoughts of animosity and detachment. He and I had made up by the end of the week; he came into the guest bedroom and said a few apologetic words. I went back to him, and my guard came down. I just wanted him to say sorry. Men never say sorry, though, typically. It makes things easier if they just apologize day one, hour one. Especially if you're married to a wife with bipolar disorder.

We usually always make up within two hours after being married two decades. But at this time I was off-kilter. By Saturday night I had not slept in two whole days, not a wink. My sedatives had run out, and my doctor's office was closed so they couldn't call in a prescription for me. Emergencies had to be taken to the hospital per the clinic's answering service. Thus one had to go to a hospital with a psychiatric ward and outpatient counseling center for help. But I didn't need counseling; I just simply needed medicines.

At 2:00 a.m. that third night of no sleep I realized I'm getting myself into dire straits. While trying to sleep next to Darrell, it dawned on me that I couldn't wait out Saturday night and then Sunday night to get sedatives Monday from the doctor. It would be very difficult to recover from that much lack of sleep and my judgment would be ruined for months. So knowing that time was running out for me and I needed to sedate myself I slipped away as quietly as possible and drove myself to the hospital ten minutes away. I wasn't going to call an ambulance and wake up everybody or have Darrell convince me not to go. He would want to handle it at home himself. But I knew if the third night was again full of insomnia, it would take months to recover. Like the doctor said, the gloves come off after night three.

In the middle of the night, I went to the ER hoping for a sedation injection. This first hospital said they didn't have a psychiatric ward. It was frustrating. After being weighed and charted and talking with a nurse then a doctor, they couldn't give me anything. Neither did they have any helpful advice. The ER doctor said he could arrange an ambulance for me to the location downtown with a psychiatric ward; and sedation could be done there.

That hospital was in the bad part of town. I wasn't going to spend another moment in an actual ward; it just brought back the memories of Canada. I just wanted an injection where I could sleep it off in the ER and be sent home later or a good amount of sedatives prescribed in the ER that I could swallow at home. If I went downtown, Darrell would also have to drive with the kids one hour to downtown the next morning. No, that wasn't practical I thought. My mind was already borderline racing and unfocused – I was trying to do a mental calculation of what made sense next. I told the doctor in the ER that I needed to go to the closer hospital twenty minutes away from here, but I'm loopy, and my mind is sped up. I told him I could drive ten residential minutes but not the interstate and that far. He went back to the fact that ambulatory transport could only be done within their health system to an affiliated hospital, not to this other hospital I was hoping to go to.

The thought of what a psychiatric ward would look downtown was daunting. I've luckily never had to see the inside of a psychiatric ward in the US. Maybe it's like a hotel depending on the part of town. Or maybe it's worse than Canada. Maybe it depends on the hospital and location within a city. Darrell never would put me in the hospital; he'd suffer through and get a homecare nurse if Bethany or Mom couldn't come in when work necessitated him back. I can count my blessings there; the majority of people don't have that luxury from a resource and capacity standpoint. What if I walked into the hospital and they committed me involuntarily? I was quickly weighing my decision whether to go to the next hospital or give up.

I told the ER doctor and nurse, "Absolutely not. I'm not going to the other hospital in your system so far away," and I knew I was too shaky to drive. It was final. They said they could not arrange ambulatory transportation for me unless it was in their health system. I was frustrated and wanted to throat punch them, but I wasn't violent by nature. I really just wanted to verbally rip into them, that would have been satisfying on some level and I was also angrily dreading they would send me a huge bill for absolutely no help. But I stayed quiet. It was useless crying over spilled milk. All I could do was to stand outside the ER again in the cool fall air, in my pajamas and braless, and call the police for a ride in the middle of the night.

I had an entire body pat down by a male police officer before getting in the car; another male officer was present during the pat down. With no bra on and in loose thin pajamas it was a horrible feeling. He was an old stout guy. If he had been movie star looking, I'd consider it totally professional and no big deal. This guy felt creepy and perverted to me. He was just doing his job though and probably somewhat uncomfortable at possible risks of any complaints I might file later. We chatted on the ride down and I shook the awkwardness of the situation off. I tried not to talk in a fast-paced manic way. I wasn't as full-blown manic as other episodes where sleeplessness ramped up for months or weeks. This was an intervention before the third night of full sleeplessness and within the seven days of the trigger of the marital conflict I'd self-created pathetically this round.

The officer dropped me off to the hospital and there I spent many hours till the first light of dawn started coming in. From one building to the next, I was shuffled this way and that way down long never ending corridors that felt cold and clammy. I walked with a blanket around my shoulders to cover the thin pajamas. Finally, they said, "We can't do anything for you unless you are about to kill yourself, we only have sedation for suicidal patients. We can just send you to the counseling office, maybe they can help." Counseling is great, but I'm a medicinal management-only case. In forty years I've been able to work out most of the therapeutic bugs I needed to work out. Maybe because I have a steady partner Darrell, and a mom who knows the illness from seeing it in her own husband – both these individuals are an important presence in realizing any early symptoms over the phone or in person. Darrell is an intelligent, gentle, intuitive person, and he gave me stability for almost two decades now. Life has been non-traumatic since leaving Canada, so I didn't need the counseling office. But the counseling office did give me something that was worth this trip. The gentleman manning the overnight booth told me to go to the pharmacy that is open twenty-four hours across the street and take melatonin and Nyquil together. He said this is the next best thing over the counter until you can call your doctor Monday for heavy prescription sedatives.

    I waited till what I thought was the more reasonable hour of 6 A.M. and called Darrell to pick me up. I was able to catch a couple hours of sleep with these over the counter items but not nearly as effective as some real medication.

    This was the turning point of awareness that a mix of sedatives I could easily have access to if planned well was the key to my recovery. At least this situation didn't morph into a long lasting and externally damaging episode. But internally within the home it had a lasting impact and sadness. A marriage that had always been smooth sailing had seen a rocky turn. It had always been satisfactory for me at least, but not so much for Darrell—he had to babysit a few episodes during our years together— and during this episode I was abrasive for the next month or two till I got my bearings. My judgment was impaired still after the week of restlessness and sleeplessness. A couple weeks after this hospital visit, we had gone on a Disney cruise we'd booked a half year prior and couldn't reschedule without losing the cruise fees. I tried to cover up being difficult with him earlier, but the trip was eclipsed by the animosities I had placed on him just weeks prior. It was hard to see each other the same way. It was hard to pretend all that strife hadn't happened. There was almost a sheepish nature to us when we looked at each other and talked to each other during that trip. It probably wasn't good for his heart as an aging man in his mid-forties to deal with drama that wasn't really surfacing from anything concrete.

I had become insecure because of the job loss, a job I'd thought I'd have till I retired and was very attached to. I had held the highest position I'd ever had in my career while at that virtual, outsourced accounting firm.

After the Disney Cruise and while still unemployed I tried breaking into separate finances with Darrell as a result of my nightclub friend advising me, and my head was too vulnerable and open to taking that advice. I was collecting unemployment money and resentful to share it with Darrell who I was at odds with as my judgment still wasn't fully back. I figured he was leaving messes around the house on purpose to demean me as though I was a maid. I wanted my own separate account and money to feel my value. This was a second time the same situation of separating finances had surfaced and it again hurt Darrell grievously. I was opening the account at a bank branch when he found me. He had tracked my location through logging in with our shared Apple ID; I had otherwise stopped location sharing from my phone number. He had walked into the bank and saw me sitting there with the banker and said pleadingly, "Please don't do this." The banker felt awkward as did I; I was embarrassed and felt exposed. I told him firmly I would see him at home later. I thought he was being domineering and trying to control me. I realized it was my same fear that I had had in the other city when I had opened an account fifteen years prior. It was the feeling that he was trying to control me and this was my way of gaining control. That first time he'd had that tear roll down his face when we discussed the bank account opening. "But I share everything with you. Why? Why this?" he had said. Here we were again in that same situation. I had taken the EAP lady's suggestion on separate finances years earlier and now I was taking the suggestion from my friend on the same matter. This suggestion wasn't my own thought; it was theirs that I'd implemented. It suited their life, not mine.

This was my sixth episode. The fifth one I hadn't mentioned yet; it was just a fleeting one inspired by my own fancy. It happened three years into my five-year job I'd just been let go from. This was a fully avoidable episode, I kind of let it happen without realizing it at the time. I had stopped taking my medicines under the belief that a study I read could mean I don't have bipolar disorder anymore. This surfaced in my mind after reading an article published by a US university related to a research study conducted on bipolar disorder and it stated that for some percentage of people the disorder does go away in one's thirties. I was hopeful and elated. I decided to go off medicines for the winter, which was the only winter I didn't put on weight because I was slightly manic and sleeping less and craving less food. I had informed my psychiatrist that I was going to test this research out. She said to stay in close contact with her if my moods change. I had been on low dosages of medicines most of my life so perhaps she felt it may be worth seeing how this pans out as well and fairly low risk.

I discontinued the medication and my appetite that usually spikes in the winter due to slight seasonal affect symptoms stayed steady this particular winter, and I wasn't craving sugar. I was elated that I didn't put on the usual ten pounds I do in the winter and then fight those ten pounds off in the summer. But the appetite subsiding was related to a slow ramp up into hypomania and without me noticing immediately. My sleep was also lessening. By month four my sleep had gone down from seven hours to only five hours nightly.

Where the realization came in that I needed my medicines finally was an incident I regret badly to this day. I had behaved erratically with Darrell, suspecting him when he was out with just his guy friends. I'd embarrassed him by showing up at their get-together late one evening, just three guys sitting there watching the tube and hanging out. A wife showing up and asking her husband to come home in a firm mean voice in front of the other guys? That's flat out embarrassing and awkward – it reflects poorly on the spousal relationship. I'm sure they were sympathetic to him and I am sure I seemed like a psychotic bitch to those men. Indeed I was off my anti-psychotic medicines for months now; hence the psychotic behavior. But maybe this happens even when someone doesn't have bipolar disorder. Perhaps I'm too hard on myself, but then again this was all avoidable had I stayed on my medicines. That wasn't the real me to behave that way even if emotionally upset with Darrell. So I went back on the pills. Darrell was livid and stopped sharing his location with me; I was unruly after all. What if I showed up when he was at a business meeting with a client? I stopped sharing my location with him, too, permanently – and got my own Apple ID so he couldn't log in as me. I did this just out of spite, but I understood why he did it on his end first. I get it. I had acted unfairly. It was too much of a chance to take; once you break that trust it's hard to earn it back.

I went through a month of talk therapy over the phone with a female therapist at Darrell's request. I just went online and subscribed to this application that matches you with a therapist virtually, and it is super cheap compared to in-office visits that schedule quite far out and are expensive. It was predominantly writing back and forth, not virtual calls except for just the initial interaction upon introduction to the therapist. Thereafter you type back and forth all month. If you want in-person calls, that costs more. I figured forget that. I'm doing this at Darrell's request, so I wasn't quite sure I was getting anything out of it anyways.

But my therapist said no, this was just a situational issue, not bipolar activity. She said people sometimes have this happen in marriages. It's not you; it's the situation. Darrell had wanted me to get the counseling because of the incident. However later I realized on my own that it was the lack of medicines creating that paranoia. Darrell had forgotten, too, that I wasn't taking them. Darrell and I are pretty devoted to each other. He's the best thing that ever happened to me. He spends every spare minute he can with me. He calls frequently while out. I'd probably be more likely to cheat on him than him on me. My libido is extremely high, maybe a side effect of being predisposed to mania. Darrell never complains about it. Infidelity would be unlikely. The best years of my life were after I married him.

Darrell and I built our dream home when we moved to the Midwest. He always wanted a custom-built home—better quality and finished appearance. But this production-builder home I truly love. It's a castle to me. Compared to anything I grew up in. We have new cars, not used. Growing up, everyone I knew could never afford new cars. Always the people we grew up around including us bought aftermarket cars.
I'd grown up differently. No one ever used car tape in the Indian community to fix things, but repairs were low priority. Plus everyone had a blue collar job and hadn't gone to college so the disposable income to buy a brand new car usually came very late in life once your children were much older.
I'm thankful for where we live. It is humbling to go to other parts of town and see cars alongside your vehicle, cars that are riddled with tape and dents with side mirrors hanging off, attached with just a wire. Many people are paycheck to paycheck in most of America; a cosmetic car repair is at the bottom of the list. Darrell grew up in India where the poverty looked different. The people there save throughout their lives to be sure there is enough for retirement in the bank as there isn't significant governmental assistance as a safety net. My husband always kept money saved up, enough for that if he lost his job tomorrow our family would get by at the same lifestyle level for six months without any assistance.
 Growing up we had a new car only once when my dad had bought one during a bipolar episode phase. If he was in his full senses he would have bought aftermarket like everyone else in

our socio-economic class. It was tragically a car he sold in a frenzy that was gone before we could even sit in it four times. It was an electric blue sedan. I can't remember what kind, but I recall its electrifying blue with acuity. How I missed that car all my childhood until I met Darrell where new was possible again. I wonder if I had been on my own if I would have engaged in spending sprees when episodic and bought cars that were above what I could afford. I shudder at thinking of a life without Darrell's sensibility. I'd like to think I would have made good decisions even without him, but weathering episodes alone could yield a frightening result. He keeps me grounded.

Darrell and Dad are such contrasts. I visited my dad a few times at the nursing home during his past five years there. For twenty-five years, he walked the streets wanting a way back into my mom's heart... sometimes attempting it violently. The restraining order was enforced a few times. I remember him trying to break the back glass sliding door with a rock in order to get inside the house. We watched out of a faraway window that was angled in the back deck's direction—Delilah, Emilia, Mom, and I. We were scared for our lives.

My mom often would want a male cousin or uncle to be around as a deterrent to Dad coming around our house. A male cousin did come to stay with us for an extended period of time while he sponsored his family and worked as a cab driver. He'd watch pornography late at night. I discovered this one time, when I got up to get a glass of water as I was uncharacteristically thirsty that particular evening.

There was a time this cousin slipped a note to my older sister that read, "I love you," which totally made her feel awkward. He moved out soon after his family came from overseas. Of course we told our mom none of this, since it somehow makes you feel incriminated as well. We also had a man my mom's age come stay with us. He was my aunt's husband, the aunt who had poisoned my dog in India. This man's goal was to come here and work, earn, and sponsor his own family from India as soon as he was eligible to do so.

It was helpful to have a man around as a deterrent to my dad trying to storm the place; but Dad was irked that a man my mom's age was living in our home. This relative was the loser type and completely flirtatious with any age female. He had this habit where he he would brush his hand on your lower backside as he passed by in the narrow hallway. Recall that other drunk, limping liar? The one that had told my X-fiancé I was into him, who I'd slapped back in India? This was his brother. It runs in the family, the perversion. My aunt's husband would make his touches look ambiguous. Keep them subtle. However they started to become habitual and obvious.

This was completely gross and inappropriate behavior, and something I complained about years later finally when I was in college, our aunt's husband took advantage of the knowledge that I smoked. He had found out from a cousin; I bet the very one who taught me and my other cousins how to smoke. So he held blackmail knowledge about me that he tried to use in his favor and control situations with.

The inappropriate behavior reached an apex of severity when my aunt's husband had started kissing me on the mouth while I was in the elevator at the courthouse waiting for my mom's settlement, and the elevator doors were shut. He was supposed to be there as a support for Mom, and it fueled my dad's anger even more that this man was present during the proceedings. That incident was too much, I felt, and it was the turning point where I whistle blew on him; he'd crossed a line. I figured it warranted the risk of being uncovered as a smoker to my mom.

I told my mom about the incident, and I also told Aunt Jennifer and their youngest brother who we'd lived with years before on the prairies. Aunt Jennifer and I had a strong bond. She'd been so proud of this straight A girl who'd gone to college. Her own adopted son had midway discontinued his power engineering certificate and instead become a plumber. She was happy for her sister's success in raising the only girl in the extended family who had been to college. She was forever on my side. She had also been the only one to support me at the time of my breakup with my first fiancé while my mom was initially disapproving of it and unsupportive. Aunt Jennifer was always in my corner.

This perverted uncle-in-law had defended himself in a primitive fashion by bringing up my smoking. I'm not sure he realized he was only damaging his position by bringing that up. The blackmail was obvious. At that time however I was taken aback and scared when he mentioned that to everyone when they had confronted him about the advance on me; I froze. But I had nothing to worry about; as logical adults Mom, Aunt Jennifer and their youngest brother saw through his tactics immediately and said, "You are out – pack your stuff. Find yourself a basement to rent."

I'm glad I stood up for myself. The knowledge of smoking uncovered to my mom was awkward for me but no one questioned me about that later. As a kid you don't do the mental calculation in your head that you shouldn't hesitate to uncover injustices even though you fear your own blackmail might be uncovered. The equation in my mind didn't make it so black and white during those younger years though. It is both strange and sad how in those adolescent years I hesitated even for a second to say something and had to dwell a bit on the blackmailing and whether I should or should not say something. Why did I tarry on it even a moment I sometimes chide myself at the memory of hesitating. To decipher beyond the manipulation took a calculated guess of weighing costs and benefits to the smoking secret that would be uncovered. It should have been more straight forward and simple that I must tell my mom what happened regardless of the blackmail. I'm glad I realized it was worth the risk of telling them, why I had to stop and think to tell them is the part I regret. I also had another worry in my mind and that was for my little sister, Emilia, that pushed me into action on uncovering this uncle-in-law's behavior. She was also living under the same roof as this man. He'd always been a perverted guy and his behavior was not going to change. I was twenty, and his advances had materialized into just a wandering caress on my side, and finally reached to a blackmailed kiss. Emilia was only thirteen. My continued indefinite silence could have had far worse repercussions.

Chapter 14

Manic Unprofessionalism

2019

After losing the long term virtual job, about two months later I did find a part-time job with a marketing company ten minutes away from home. It seemed like a dream job as it was close to home, part time, and just a single company's set of books instead of the multi-client juggling environment I'd always been in. However a few months in, I realized the CFO was of a sketchy character and not transparent. Everyone rumored she was having the owner's baby which is a separate can of worms but what I struggled with was the relevant matter of when she told me she was going to transfer funds to another bank account so the owner wouldn't see it in the usual bank he logs into. This was for the purpose of hiding an incoming half-million-dollar payment to be received in the next week from a large customer for the reason that she was worried that the owner would spend it on other things and not the main operational costs. She said he was going to make a large real estate purchase for the company that was completely unnecessary. Truly I noticed he had ostentatious behavior with spending that was not judicious at all, however what the CFO was doing was evasive.

I had assumed indeed it was going to go to another company account. But I'm not sure if the money would end up there or elsewhere. Compounded with her non-transparent behavior was that she was a highly toxic fixture in this environment, and operations folks were scared of her. I'd been in many environments and seen healthy dynamics and then seen people who pulled others from climbing the corporate ladder, hoarding knowledge to themselves. I'd seen it all by now. I had started to finally recognize some of this behavior by this stage in my career. I was never good at reading people. It has taken me a lifetime to recognize some things aren't as they seem. Maybe that is because I am a talker and not so much a listener. But listening attentively is a skill I need to develop fast and remain consistent with. Listen in order to understand, not listen in order to just respond. Those who listen can perceive and understand more about the people they navigate around. Darrell is a listener, and I like men who don't talk much. I feel they are better situated as they observe, assess and are careful that any jargon doesn't unnecessarily come out of their mouths that can be lies or over telling of truths. Beware of men who talk too much is a saying I've heard more than once in various ancient literary works.

Those who showed this CFO opposition, she finagled out of the company and was able to get those people fired as she had the boss's ear. I had a dotted line to the owner; she had a straight line. She was also very aggressive in changing revenue numbers for the bank lending reports that were sent monthly so the loans wouldn't become callable. At this point I figured I was getting that fraud anxiety again. That was not good. Also there were rumors of drugs in the bathroom and accusations on who left them there, there was finger pointing between the top ranks. There was shouting in the daily morning management meetings. It was becoming quite the dramatic scenery. I didn't need another episode to come on by sticking up for transparency in reporting to the owner and trying to weather the office drama and politics. As the AICPA had said a year prior, "Just leave the problem company if you ever get into that uncomfortable area again. That is what people have to do" So I took that advice this time as my paramount concern was the incoming funds re-routing and misleading debt covenant disclosures. It wasn't a good environment anyways and it would take an act of God to change the situation and make it a healthy work place.

I resigned without notice. I had a phone exit interview and told the CEO and the owner all that was going on. It was the right thing to do on transparency. I later heard from one of the operations people who sat beside the CFO—he was my desk buddy—that the owner had immediately called her after talking with me. I just rolled my eyes at that; maybe they were in bed together. I had never wanted to believe the office gossip. As an owner I'd think a judicious process would be taken, an in-person meeting, a forensic audit, a consultation with your CEO. Nope. Not in this case. It was like a husband turning to casually ask his wife, what are you doing?

I had Darrell as a safety net; I always did. It made me perhaps more careless in a way. If I was a single mom supporting a family, even with bipolar disorder, I'd be more on the straight and narrow at my jobs and stick to it and attempt to weather through any stresses. Perhaps I'd stay out of trouble more. Does trouble find me or do I create trouble or do I just grab passing trouble?

In tandem with this part-time marketing company job, I'd taken another part-time job doing taxes from home for the same multi-state CPA firm I had worked a standalone busy season for back in 2011. When I resigned the marketing company I requested more hours from the CPA firm and they were happy to give them to me.

Finally I had resigned from an employer and it was nice that it was not an involuntary dismissal like all the other times. This was completely my choice. Wow. I'd done it. But my resignation was strangely not without its mental anguish either. It stayed with me a whole month. It was a shakeup I hadn't expected. I told my friend Marina I felt like such a lightweight for having it disturb me that way. She said, "Don't be so hard on yourself. You thought there was a future there for you to grow into a controller role, then a CFO, it's natural to feel the distress of a hope you had to walk away from."

I was in a stupor for a month. Darrell surprised me with taking me out to a movie. He's never for surprise gifts. That's when I had the awareness that I needed to pull it together immediately. I was starting to be on the borderline of becoming a nuisance to him to have to babysit again – this was possibly my harsh and overly critical perception of the situation. He never alluded to this at all, but I didn't want to risk wearing out his efforts to bring me back into my own. I dusted myself off after that affectionate surprise evening he gave me and I forced myself out of my stupor. I put my energy back into looking for my next job after this busy season stint ended with the CPA firm.

We went to Las Vegas with the kids and also to the Grand Canyon before I started my next job. It was at the tail end of busy season and I'd asked the company if I could have time away and do spring break with the kids – which for CPAs spring break is a novelty seldom experienced as it usually occurs during tax crunch time. Since it was a fairly no strings attached contract employment with unpaid vacation they approved the time away and I didn't check email while out which was very liberating. With all my past employers I would always check emails and respond to priority ones; I never liked coming back to surprises. I'd also always check emails for the additional purpose to not create a situation where someone has to unnecessarily spin their wheels in your absence on a client you know in and out where a quick call, text or email can alleviate the issue that would otherwise take hours for someone to figure out. I've changed my philosophy now though; family first and work a far second. Jobs come and go, family doesn't. You only get that time once with your kids while they are dependent on you. That quality time invested goes a long way later in life in terms of how connected and emotionally invested the children remain with their parents.

I was looking forward to my next venture in private company accounting as I'd finally broken away from public accounting and its multi-client facing environment.

I interview phenomenally well. I had several offers, including one from a CPA recruiting firm that was to build their business development with C-suite folks on benched consultants. They had reached out to me on LinkedIn, no doubt seeing a CPA profile with so many job hops and likely ascertaining I was not the best fit for traditional accounting work.

After my final private accounting job loss I'll go into shortly, I took the entire LinkedIn profile down and deactivated it completely. It looked like an embarrassing checkerboard of jobs by the end of 2019 and I'd started to slice and dice to reduce it to a few employers but LinkedIn becomes an open playground of judging those gaps for everyone to see and collaborate on. It was a Jenga puzzle of trying to figure out what to keep on there – I figured to just reduce my digital footprint and take my hoppy resume off the grid completely.

Becoming an accounting recruiter was a refreshing prospect. I'd talked to the recruiting company and they'd made me an offer to become their 'client', not 'candidate', facing recruiter. However I took the pragmatic road of accepting an accounting lead position at a local waste management company just nine minutes away from home, and for the first time ever in my career, almost twenty years by this point, I was going to hit a six-figure salary.

I loved being in the office again and getting dressed up, fully corporate style. I'd grown up working high-end fashion and then later working in the downtown of glamorous, glitzy corporate Vancouver. It was fun to coordinate the day's outfit in just three minutes in the morning; I had an acute eye for fashion still. Starting at an upper end retail fashion store in high school gave me a certain knack for classy attire.

The office ladies were always complimenting me periodically when I passed by, as no one dressed that way. I took fashion risks too—vibrant colors, unique styles, and always tasteful. Never was the clothing skanky. People can see through that type of dress in corporate America – as tasteless. Indeed wear what makes you happy, but also be fully aware of your professional presence and its perception.

I was genuinely happy and good at what I did on the accounting side; my confidence was back within a month. The confidence helped me with acuity in other areas of life too. It helped in areas like domestic matters, financial decisions, mothering decisions, conversing with my spouse on complicated matters and getting buy-in from others to do something a certain way.

This company's management team saw my experience with a Multinational accounting firm and seventeen years behind me (I had trimmed off the internship and Canadian work so it wasn't showing a 20 year span anymore) and they had a lot of faith in me. I was doing a great job and truly knocking it out of the park. The past Accounts Receivable where money is tied up with customers not paying, of over $800,000, I had been able to collect on. The previous person in the position, a controller who wasn't very good at what he did, had never thought to try to follow up on past collections. Or maybe later I realized he hadn't had the bandwidth. I was meticulous and tenacious with phone calls to customers and emails, they wanted me off their back. So checks and wires would come in during the first couple months of my employment there so they wouldn't continually be harassed in a professional manner. I was a super star to management, facilitating cash flow by accelerating past collections.

In a small company you wear many hats, and the list of responsibilities keeps growing. I wasn't a lawyer, but the management team added contracts analysis to my plate. They didn't understand accounting and legal areas were their own separate specialties and required their own bandwidth. I was scrubbing vendor contractors and doing procurement analysis. Then there was the compounding factor of a whole subset of customers who wanted to use their own legal contracts and not ours. Those were increasingly difficult to scrub. But I had to scrub all types of them – whether these were internally drafted contracts on a standard template that had to be overhauled, or external contracts with vastly different jargon and up to 60 pages of legalities from another customer or vendor's legal counsel. This task was something that someone solely is designated to do and spend their entire full time hours administrating such a task in a company with this volume of activity. Larger companies have armies devoted to just this task.

    Understand one can do either depth or volume, not both.

    My workload became heavier with large multi-million dollar project accounting and revenue recognition as this contract came in from new customers overseas. I had to manage invoicing and keep track of purchase orders in supplier portals to deal with paying customers that were SEC level giants and had their own systems every vendor had to adjust to. It was becoming a nightmare and not scalable for one person anymore. Revenue invoicing was its own ball of wax that took a few days of the cycle itself.

    I was recognized for customer sales collections but also for being judicious about what vendors got paid and which were delayed on the expense side of the business. The previous controller was arbitrary with money and not focusing on when cash flow was needing to be tightened and which vendors to pay when. Part of this indifference was that they had received a large cash cushion that floated the company for years. They had received both a large bank loan and huge chunk of investor financing years ago, and the controller budgeted the usage, but now we were close to zero with little funds left and the existing bank was skeptical about lending. A new banking relationship was being vetted as the current one refused lending additional funds to the company. Investors were not enthusiastic about funding more into the company either. It's a whole different monster when you have to do cash management on a daily and weekly basis to make company ends meet. There were a host of daily tasks introduced trying to budget and meet payroll and vendor needs. I'm someone who hasn't revved up in my career slowly to a sustained eighty- to ninety- hour work week. Investment banking in the early years is like that I heard. But maybe folks are younger and right out of the gate are groomed for those rigorous hours. Or maybe it's my bipolar diagnosis that doesn't allow me to sustain that schedule on low sleep levels.

CPAs work sixty- to eighty-hour work weeks in public accounting's tax and audit busy season and know it will end after a three month period. We know it isn't going to go on without a break. CPAs who work in SEC companies with one company's set of books sometimes work for ten months or more at this same sustained level of hours, hitting ninety hours in certain situations especially around an acquisition of a firm. Perhaps again it's in the early grooming or a slow build up of stamina over the years to sustain that schedule and be able to keep up with it without burnout. These people have trained for the marathon and are conditioned differently; they deal with the load and life goes on. A bipolar mind like mine caves and folds. Or perhaps I went from zero to sixty in too short a time and there was no three month window where I knew there was light at the end of the tunnel. I didn't know where in this tunnel I was and how far it stretched.

I had worked from home in my pajamas for five years. And now I was working eighty to ninety hours a week.

I went from a consistent, small private company schedule as a generalist accounting lead to having procurement duties on my plate. There were many ramp-ups to every faucet of my job during my time there and new ones developing daily. The revenue cycle was getting complex and there were bank audits and tax agency audits I shouldered solely as well.

This waste management company's board had demanded reports monthly by the 9th business day. The financials were to be put on a series of spreadsheets that a consultant had built for them, which were extremely clunky and part hard key and part formula driven, with excel IF statements and pivot table data feeds. It was both financial and accounting data, with budgets and forecasts into the future. There was a whole element of financial analyst work to this reporting, not just accounting. Before me the financials were always sent in advance of the 20th calendar day. I was expected to do it in less than half that time now. I had migrated the company's accounting system to completely new and different software that would integrate with the new payroll system and work better with the new bank. They figured there had been some efficiencies I had gained so I should be able to do closings in less than half the time as my predecessor. This was an oversimplified assumption on their end.

The CFO owned this board report task for a while, where she did the modeling and spread-sheeting. She had a heavy finance background but not so much accounting in her previous years. I was open in the interview about how finance wasn't in my wheelhouse. She said she'd teach me. They were paying me a lot of money. I thought, okay, let's do this. But then this deliverable became my responsibility entirely, by month four. I struggled to keep up.

I was starting another slow manic phase, climbing that manic bell curve up its left side.

My days started roughly at 6:50 a.m. and went to 8:30 p.m. That was Monday through Friday, with Saturday and Sunday another eight to ten hours each day. There were some nights where I worked till midnight.

The wheels started to come off of my performance. Board reports were late the month I was let go. Junior staff in operations had gone to Costco with the company credit card they requested for an evening office party, and their card wasn't functional. I had been asked hurriedly by our secretary to help them, as she had to watch the front desk. I had a lot to do, but figured I can run out within the hour during lunch and get it done as Costco is only eight minutes away from the office.

I ran out in that lunch hour and was out one hour and twelve minutes. I backed into this time later. During my firing meeting, the CFO said:

1) I was unprofessional.
2) Board reports were late.
3) I had gone to Costco on my job time.

I was choked. This was told to me only when I prodded her for reasons. Otherwise she was not going to give me any explanations. I exclaimed to the CFO that Costco was during my lunch break plus it was for company supplies for the office party during that particular evening on our premises. I reminded the CFO we were doing it on site under budget this time instead of at a venue, thus the trip to the store. Management had been so happy about the money saving for the office party, at least up until now.

Yes, the board reports were late, something I kept her fully apprised of with step-by-step progress updates. But the "unprofessional" comment confused me. I kept thinking about it for a month afterward, trying to figure out what had happened.

I keep myself pretty regulated, since I have this illness, with self awareness and constant re-evaluating of the perception of my image at all times. But I was starting a manic episode induced by low sleep that commenced almost two months prior. Maybe I had slipped somewhere and didn't keep the poise up.

There was so much work in the office that Maddy and Hudson would sit in the dark playing on their iPads when I came home in the evening, if Darrell was working late. They would let themselves in and not switch on the lights or remember to eat until we got home.

It was winter already and the sun went down early. Darrell was single parenting those last two months of my job at the waste management company. He took care of the kids, meals, dishwasher, laundry, and house in general while running an entire division at work. Darrell wanted me to succeed. I wanted me to succeed. This was my first six-figure job.

My mom called that November while I was at work, a week before I was let go. Mom had told me, "I think Maddy is going into depression, Alayna. I face-timed with her earlier today. She's so quiet and stopped responding to Izzy." Izzy was Delilah's daughter. Izzy was sixteen, and Maddy was fourteen. They would often exchange social media messages and sometimes live video call each other. My mom had seen depression; she had felt depression herself. And Mom wanted to intervene the second she thought something might be going downhill.

I went into one of the conferences room while having this conversation with Mom. It had glass walls and otherwise it was an open office environment, all conference alcoves and meeting rooms were just glassed in, no privacy. I turned myself to the wall and cried after hanging up. As silently as possible I sobbed, the tears ran down my face and my nose was red, and I used my blouse's sleeve to wipe a badly running nose. I then darted back to my desk before I could meet eyes with anyone. Later I ran to the bathroom to get cleaned up, which was further away down the hall. Why didn't I see that a job, even a six-figure one, wasn't worth jeopardizing my children's health? I should have put in my two week's notice or told the CFO that I have no more capacity in terms of trying to meet deadline after deadline, I just can't with it and need a few days off. Or that we need to outsource the routine duties absolutely now (something I'd requested already but the CFO had dismissed the idea). Darrell was doing fine at work – I could leave the job, but it was a lot of money so very difficult to give up on.

It came back to me, the unprofessional event that likely sealed it for me in terms of a firing.

There was an Operations Lead guy who was very friendly with me and helpful to everyone, almost to a fault. But he was also very opportunistic and knew how to play the game. He tried many times to exploit financial information and gauge some sense of how the company was doing overall. Everyone at the company was concerned over the years that financially something was going downhill.

Accounting and human resource functions must remain tight-lipped at all times, regardless of friendships with other departments. I deflected repeated questions from this Operations Lead person over the months I was there, but in month six and seven, I was climbing the manic hill. I was not so tight-lipped anymore and my judgment was starting to slide from me.

The Friday before I was fired, in the open office environment where at least five others sat, the Operations Lead asked me pointedly, "So why is the board here so often?"

Instead of quarterly the board of investors who is above the management team was indeed here monthly now as of the last few months. Investors had skin in the game. Losses were high. Concerns ran even higher for those who had invested heavily. And not just the Operations Lead but other employees had started to ask carefully placed questions of me to try to get a feel for the company's health and if they should be looking. I was always tight-lipped. No one had braved asking in such an overt public fashion until now.

I was already somewhat manic and not discreet enough. In my usual humorous fashion, I said to the Lead in response to why they are always here, "Because we're their bitch." I continued to sip my coffee from the company logo-etched mug.

Everyone had chuckled in the area. But I'm sure it made at least one of them uneasy enough to go to HR. I finally realized this massive error after I stayed at home, had time to decompress and regain my balance after a boatload of sedatives. I concluded this comment was likely what sealed my termination. That was the unprofessionalism that made its way to management, and by the following Friday, I was fired. Management had taken it personally. I was a high functioning bipolar person who didn't seem off kilter or unstable in the least, it wasn't entirely obvious like it had once been at my first job I'd lost at the Multinational CPA firm when I was post partum with Maddy long ago. In that situation clearly people knew something was amiss with my rapid pressured speech that ran up tangents. In contrast to that job, at this waste management company I appeared highly functional and coherent still, thus management didn't think twice before pulling the plug. I likely just appeared to be a smart mouth to them. When I called my physiatrist and told her about losing this job she made me aware of the fact that often people appearing highly functional in the workplace are terminated without a second thought whereas if very obvious behavioral instability is witnessed then the employer is more likely to engage in due process.

The CFO had called me into a conference room on Friday at 4:30 p.m. I'd already sent her the board reports for the month and completed the bank audit successfully. That last week when I'd get an email, I'd hear her computer make a sound every time too. It crossed my mind that it couldn't be a coincidence. She was on my 'bcc' likely and incoming box monitoring. Also, the screen started slowing and getting choppy with my mouse, having that slowdown freeze-frames look. The thought crept into my mind more than a few times that my computer was being monitored live by the remote IT firm. No, it couldn't be though. I'm doing great here. It's not surveillance; it's in my head. It was already difficult enough to focus with the mania starting and being low on sleep for weeks now. Tasks were taking longer. I was falling behind. As an internal service provider to other departments, I never had the luxury to put earphones in as people needed to tap me on the shoulder for things frequently. Something or other always needed to be ordered, a requisition for this or that, payroll questions, etc. There was always infinitely distracting noise even on a baseline day. With an unfocused mind developing, it became exponentially difficult to work in such an environment.

I wager upper management saw it as a grave insult to be called someone's bitch. It became personal for them. The CFO would just likely outsource my position to the current CPA firm provider and try to get by. I was a loose cannon. I couldn't be kept on staff where already folks were nervous about the company situation and trying to prod information frequently.

I'd made that remark on Friday, and it had been seemingly benignly in my bipolar brain, one that didn't need a further dwelling on in terms of any regrets saying it or analyzing for repercussions. The following Tuesday before my firing, I had the desperation to discuss with the CEO that I was overworked. I was working all weekend, every weekend. As of the recent weekend after processing many tasks I was looking at Six

Sigma-type remedies to help the company turn its failing situation around. I had worked every day for a straight nine weeks. We were about to start to incur more debt and go into a daily cash management situation shortly. I was going to discuss Six Sigma approaches with management later when they next could have a meeting with me. I had sent some weekend emails to invite management to help brainstorm an approach for profitability as I'd gathered valuable insight to cost cutting areas and with being in accounting gained an A – Z perspective of the parts of the business that weren't speaking to one another, the departmental breakages, inefficiencies, and wasted money. On Tuesday I told the CEO that I had asked the CFO about hiring a clerk to help me, and that she had said "No" earlier that day. The CFO had told me the new person requisitioned in our department would be helping her on the finance side, not accounting.

The CEO told me he was glad I went to him and to always consider it an open office environment. He kept looking at his watch during our brief few minutes of discussion in the side room, as he had a dinner meeting with the board that evening again. That Friday he gave the longest dirtiest look over the cubicles to me, and I was confused. It was the kind of look that cannot be mistaken for any other kind of look; the glare that lasts a good five seconds and is full of animosity. It was truly awkward and a dark look you squirmed under.

To this day, I earnestly wish I could have told that CEO about my mental breakdown I was having. I wish I could have told him that I had bipolar disorder and was buckling under the pressure. Perhaps he would have understood; perhaps he would have had logical compassion. He was a level headed genuine guy at least from what I could assess over those months I was there. But maybe I couldn't have told him. Maybe I'd be on the radar for replacement after a year or so even if all was well till then. Maybe they would be nervous about the next downturn in my psychology.

I was fired by the CFO with a second person listening over the speaker phone from the Professional Employer Organization

(PEO). The PEO was our payroll company. It was the lady from our PEO service that was the witness to the HR meeting. The HR director that was an internal employee to our organization was not present, only the contracted PEO representative assigned to the waste management company's file was filling in. The HR director had already left for the day. The firing was preplanned, days in advance I'm guessing, but likely it took them a couple of days to corroborate the complaints from staff if my speculation was correct on what the main cause was—that unprofessional comment.

    I'd like to think this HR director didn't want to be there to fire me; the HR director and I were friends in the way workplace colleagues can become buddies to a certain degree. We would grab a bite to eat together at a restaurant or bring lunch back to our desks sometimes and chat all the while. I would share best practices I saw at other firms. But Human Resources is a silo, and they have to work in a silo always. Their alliance is to the company. I'd like to think the HR director had skipped that meeting on purpose. Maybe she understood the hours and breakdown I was having silently as I sat diagonal to her daily. Or maybe she really had to pick up her car from the shop that afternoon. She had been there till the afternoon but then left early for that errand. A firing usually means the HR director is there with the other management, come heck or high water – for a critical event like that.

    She had left in the afternoon. I was there alone with the CFO, in shock at losing my six-figure job I'd cherished and had busted doing now for months at the detriment of my children. The CFO didn't let me touch anything other than allow me to grab my purse from the drawer, and she was watching carefully. The CFO had even put my coat in the waiting area before she'd fired me. It was insulting and degrading when I looked for it on the stand next to our set of desks and it wasn't there and she informed me she had moved it already.

    I never sued any of the companies that terminated me. Although it crossed my mind, a few times, on the grounds of medical issue discharge. My behavioral issues were never given due process – but I never told any of them either about my condition. Would they have not fired me had I told them at some point while everything was kosher that I have this condition and need an accommodation at times? Should I have said disabled on my applications? Would they feel resentful if I had told them only after the application process? Do I need a special accommodation? Nowadays there are a lot of electronic application questions on your status and if you need accommodations due to disability, of any kind. I always say there is no disability, but I don't know if that would ever become an issue ... if I have a breakdown and an employer knows it was a pre-existing condition I didn't mention I need an accommodation for; maybe that's grounds for dismissal immediately as you are basically lying to the employer when getting hired that I'll never need an accommodation for disability that was there to begin with. It's a bit of a dilemma figuring out if and when to disclose the illness, ever.

    I was in an employment-at-will State. You can be terminated by an employer for any reason based on the state's employment laws, other than if discriminatory. I wasn't about to pursue a false minority woman case. That would be a total lie. None of these companies ever discriminated against me based on race or gender. I was a pretty cooperative and agreeable team player. I was a very emotionally regulated individual; I had a lot to hide. I was never too happy or too sad. I was constantly self-monitoring and likeable. I was successful as an organizational unit when my mind didn't get away from me. I never tried to sue, although I was frustrated as heck with each company. I was too scared to uncover my bipolar diagnosis. I wanted to continue practicing as a CPA without a tarnished public reputation. If you go into a lawsuit against an employer, that's a history you don't want. Especially if there is no settlement that's enough to retire on. It's so much harder to find a local job if you become notorious that way. You've shot yourself in the foot financially if all you've walked away with is a couple years of wages as a settlement.

Losing the waste management company job was as blessing in disguise, yet another setback that somehow worked out for the better in the long run. I was fighting not to get a bout of depression that following month in December. The job I had lost in November was one where I'd earned money at the highest rate I'd ever been able to for myself. I felt my confidence ebb away, and I was desperately warding off insecurities. I'd already screwed up my marriage once during the previous September when I'd lost the work-from-home job. That time I'd ruined for us what was a once-in-a-lifetime Disney cruise that was overshadowed by Darrell's and my only brutal fight in seventeen years. But I hope overcoming that strife made us stronger, those we made up from always. Like a wound that heals afterward, the tissue is stronger that heals it over. I reminded myself over and over again daily: don't repeat the mistake of getting into an unnecessary brawl that is completely self-instigated.

Don't do it again, Alayna. Don't become psychotic with Darrell again.

So I resolved to stay content as a homemaker. I told myself it takes nine months to make a habit. Stick to it, things will get better. My children had literally jumped up and down with joy when they found out mom was fired and back home again full time and they begged me to not go back to work ever again. Maddy told me when I told her I need to find something again eventually though: "Mom can you work from home again like you did before? I like seeing you when I get off the bus."

I visited my family back home during Christmas break, with Darrell beside me who is my rock. I stay more even keel with him by my side when I go back to Vancouver where there is a bustle of memories. I can visit Darrell's family on the US West Coast and be totally unfazed by manic tendencies. Vancouver was different, the place of nightmares but also beautiful mountains and ocean. There were some good memories, although they are eclipsed with mostly bad ones. This past December I'd finally made peace with everything and the emotions never came in like a freight train as they usually did. I spent time with my dad, we celebrated his and my birthdays together with side by side cakes at Delilah's house. Our birth month and day were less than a week apart.

I saw my dad in the nursing home again in December, visiting him a few times and we'd brought him home to Delilah's for the birthday celebration as well. This time I didn't leave the nursing home crying uncontrollably like the last couple times I was there visiting him in years past. Darrell was with me. In those previous instances by the time I got back to the parking lot, I would have tears rolling down my eyes and while driving all the way back to Mom's house those tears continued. I was dangerously driving with limited view because of the watery eyes. I would mop the tears up quickly so no one saw. If my family saw they'd think I was having an episode and tell me not to go visit Dad again the next day, out of concern for me. My time with him was precious; I couldn't screw that up.

Delilah and I have had the discussion over the phone years ago. Do we love him? Or do we just feel sorry for him? And the reality is it is just sympathy. Pure sympathy and then some empathy. Not a deep seeded love. It makes me sad, but I cannot bring myself to feel moved by him out of love.

I had a reoccurring task on my calendar to call Dad; it reminded me to call him weekly. Yet my mom, I call daily without a reminder. I wait for it to be 9:05 a.m. (PST), when she'll be awake and has had a few minutes to situate. We moved all our love over to our mom, us three girls; there was not much left in Dad's share. Life had done that to us. I prepare myself for the day he won't be here any longer. People with vascular dementia only live five to eight years after initial diagnosis. I sincerely hope I feel less regret and guilt when that happens, and thus I call him to alleviate that burden of guilt that may be felt eventually. I visit him. I'm not propelled to out of love for him. I'm propelled out of obligation and easing my already bipolar mind that one day I might not live with any regrets when he is no longer here; regrets that I didn't reach out to him. Perhaps the shadow of love I only fleetingly feel at times stem from those few childhood memories of him pushing us on the swings or becoming a play horse we could sit on. I could not feel sorry for him on the subject of him having a mental illness for he had the opportunity many times to get help from his loved ones but he stayed difficult and abusive and threw out his life himself. I wish he had been open to help long ago and had stayed on medication and sought counseling back in the 80s when he was first diagnosed. Those tender childhood years would have looked markedly different. Mom's life wouldn't have been so scarred either.

One of my Indian friends, Marina, is the only person outside the family who knows of my ailment. My husband had my mom tell Marina a year prior, during that Disney Cruise time frame episode. It was initiated from a safety perspective to protect me. When my mom told me she would tell her, I told her not to and that I'd tell Marina myself. I wasn't an invalid. I hard lined that fact with Darrell and Mom.

Marina was my female confidante. I talked to her more often and texted with her more often than I did Delilah and Emilia, my own sisters. Marina was in the same time zone as me and in the finance industry. She was dealing with bipolar disorder in her spouse as well. We had a connection, she and I. It was helpful for her to know the inside of a bipolar mind. I was a highly functional bipolar individual who was successful in keeping myself coherent and connected 97.5% of my life and episode free. It was mutually beneficial, the knowledge sharing. I would never dare talk directly to her spouse who was dealing with bipolar disorder about our ailment, although it would have been lovely to. This individual was in denial of his illness. Marina was dear to me in that she was on the same wavelength as me, being ingrained in the finance industry for 20 years. We'd both earned our stripes in different ways. She was from India too. She went through the same cultural pressures in the younger years as me, and now like me was able to shake those pressures off completely to acclimate entirely to the North American way of living. Plus Marina was raised in Canada. That was an instant connection for us initially. She led the book club I had joined through another friend's suggestion who'd said I'd really like Marina and relate to her.

Marina gave me praise at times, that I'd shy away from. I tend to self doubt a lot. But perhaps it's the safety feature in my mind not to attain any grandiosity that my bipolar mind could grab onto, obsess, and fixate over. Letting strong praise go to my head may put me on a quick upswing of excitement unnecessarily.

That last month at the waste management company, Marina had said in retrospect, "Alayna, you were like a freight train crashing that I couldn't look away from; this job loss was for the better. Don't feel bad for yourself that it happened."

Another girlfriend told me something when I was at the bottom of this jobless insecurity pit. "Your profession is for you; you are not for your profession." She'd lost a job, and those were her father's words of wisdom. Powerful words. It's just a financial loss. Why does it feel so much like an identity loss to me however? This is a natural state to be in, I researched this to a tedious degree. Many out there feel that way, just as I did. Yet it doesn't give us closure or comfort right away, this fact that massive amounts of people go through the same thing we just did. The job loss still ends up miring a lot of us into depression. But I continue to try to memorize the fact that it's just a financial loss, and a temporary one. The loss is absolutely not a reflection on you – don't perceive yourself as a faulty or worthless person. The way we internalize things sometimes, we become our own biggest enemy.

Be kind to yourself.

Sometimes I think of when I will retire, and those golden years. Is it easier to go first? So you don't have to bear the suffering of losing your soul mate? I don't want to live with my kids and their families. There is always that level of formality to maintain while living with in-laws that goes both ways on the endless gridlock of discomfort. I don't want to live in a nursing home. I don't even have long-term care insurance yet, and the more you age the more expensive it gets. I don't want to lose Darrell early and be alone.

But if that happens I want to be mentally prepared and a game plan. I want to co-live in a retirement community. If Darrell is no longer here then I would not want to live alone but would want to co-live with a girlfriend or sister.

The loneliness of old age is stagnating and horrifying, and the mental regression into Alzheimer's is worse – the onset of which sometimes comes on with the imminent solitude of living alone.

Darrell and I have friends of the same sex and other couples we hang out with as a pair. They say if you ever commiserate about your marriage, never do it with someone of the opposite sex; it's an exploitive area. It's letting the devil in the backdoor. Commiserate, if you have to, but with a person of the same gender. Or better yet commiserate back with your other half. One will see better results with their marriage if one goes to the source of the conflict. When I look to the older years there needs to be preparedness on my part not to be vulnerable to men or women and build a careful trusted circle.

In Eastern cultures you live with your parents until you are married, and then they live with you later upon their retirement; such is the circle of Eastern life. Times change, and there is a greater independence, options, and financial security for elderly people. Some don't need to necessarily rely on a joint-family system and be forced under a one-roof setting with multiple children's families co-living together. As a generation, for the most part, born and raised in America, we are so much more mobile than those who migrated here before us in their golden years.

I often wonder what will happen with my bipolar situation in older years and will it look different. The following is helpful to understand the additional complexity of the illness faced in the geriatric years.

Bipolar Disorder in later life is a complex and confounding neuropsychiatric syndrome with diagnostic and therapeutic challenges. Complicating the clinician's approach to treatment of older patients with BD is the paucity of controller pharmacological studies in this age group.
—— www.psychiatrictimes.com (December 1, 2007 article by Nhi-ha Trinh MD)

The fact that the geriatric years muddy the waters in terms of what is related to bipolar disorder versus what is another health condition is disheartening and unsettling. I was hoping as I continue to grow I would have this illness on lock. I have some anxieties over getting into my golden years and being without my loved ones if I were to outlive them. At the edge of my mind I am afraid that my bipolar ailment might take me by surprise in those years where elders are susceptible to dementia. I continue to force myself to focus on a diet and exercise regimen in order to have healthy geriatric years. Darrell's mom always said what you eat in your 30s you will feel the impact of in your 50s. So I continue to try not to neglect my physical health although mental health becomes the overriding concern mostly.

Mentally I worry I will rapid cycle daily or from month to month. I worry I may fall into an episode without stabilizing. I worry I may not have the support of a trusted circle of loved ones who would be brutally honest with me about my mood and one that would monitor me frequently until my self-awareness comes back. I think at times perhaps I should plan for having a pet to help ward off possible depression, but I'm historically on the manic side so that might not help. A pet's excitement might actually add to the mania.

Perhaps a grey haired manic woman can play the old senile card, and I'll just blend in. To blend in is a luxury I've always wanted. I've yearned for a permanent cure to bipolar disorder. But I try to remember, there are worse ailments the doctors are focusing on to cure.

I read that menopause for women with bipolar disorder is more challenging as there is a greater susceptibility of mood changes during that stage. I can only hope for the best and plan for the worst. I have started writing down and sharing this risk and concern with loved ones. I hope my being fully aware of the higher risk as I enter that stage of life in this next decade will be adequate enough in setting up my success to reach out for help and consult with my doctor proactively in order to survive through it episode free.

Chapter 15

Hopeful Outlook

I find with age I am controlling the episodes better where I can deflect them from being extremely severe, prolonged, or requiring hospitalization. However I do notice I am now showing the pattern of struggling to stave off an oncoming episode more frequently – although they are less severe their possibility tends to creep up more often. Sometimes I wonder if my bipolar disorder is worsening with age in that it seems like you are more susceptible to fall into an episode frequently, always at the cusp of an impending upswing or downswing. I feel I have the illness under control as I can remedy my insomnia immediately with a repertoire of medicines. Insomnia is my main trigger to the mania. However I feel like I more frequently have to keep it under control. I contemplate if age renders various medicinal adjustments necessary, like an increase to dosages, but I'm not sure. Or is it that life has more responsibilities to juggle and higher stakes along the way that burden you and create triggering stressors? I'm certain there may be at least two major factors where bipolar disorder seems to worsen with age:

1) Externally created factor: Additional levels of responsibilities in life's areas like family, work, etc. where stress compounds

2) Internally created factor: Enhanced awareness of one's diagnosis with constant re-evaluation if psychosis is starting (over-diagnosing thoughts and feelings)

The statistics for people with bipolar disorder in terms of average episodes during a lifetime has me worried and not overly confident that all my episodes are behind me now as I've had six through this point in life.

The John Hopkins Guide cites:

Nearly all patients who have one manic episode will have another; the number of manic episodes varies from person to person, but the average number of episodes a patient will have in a lifetime is nine. Some patients have rapid cycling - with four or more manic or depressive episodes in a year.

https://www.hopkinsguides.com/hopkins/view/Johns_Hopkins_Psychiatry_Guide/ 787045/all/Bipolar_I_Disorder

I was at four major episodes and two mini episodes already, and deflected the seventh episode after taking many sedatives and shutting off the workflow valve entirely. At this point I hope I'm done having episodes, but the possibility of one is always top of mind on an almost daily basis. It seems life continues to have added responsibilities and worries in its various faucets so where there were only a handful of linear worries in the younger years, now they offshoot into many prongs and are numerous in these older years when you are monitoring your teenagers, balancing many other responsibilities as well as managing things that come up unexpectedly. Sometimes it feels like the onset of bipolar disorder is right around the corner if you stop monitoring it for a day as you age – but I think it's the external factors that change and pressure the internal illness, not just an age related chemical change in the mind or body that needs adjustment. The known exception being menopause of course, that is definitely an internal chemical force that will affect the brain.

When life events happen, it's destabilizing for us. In most of my episodes, a job loss or stress during the job destabilized me. Or it was postpartum that also did me in, with the job and combined care of young children as a compounding factor.

Historically I had fixated and obsessed on some job incident or become overworked, and then the loss of identity caused issues later during the unemployment periods. Tears are for tragedy and family, not for the things that happens at work. I rack my brain each time there is a job loss. What is my pattern? I have another twenty-five years before I retire. The contract job is working well for now. I hope I can keep it. I'm tucked away at home which is safe for my mind in some regards. I started this work just recently. I resigned one work from home place after six weeks of being there as it was a sweatshop environment I was quickly realizing, and I figured once I burnt out after a few months I'd be too tired to look elsewhere and making mistakes and eventually would be let go involuntarily. So I jumped ship early to the contract work I'd been offered at the same time as when I'd taken the sweatshop job.

If I have a life event and destabilize, I can camouflage some of the symptoms and erratic behavior because I'm working from home. Also I can work later in the week with a few days off if I need to catch up on sleep. What the future holds I'm not sure, but I've learned a lot from the past and hope to continually grow and be able to apply the knowledge from the years behind me. I think of a future for my children where Darrell and I can continually provide the stability they need. This genetic predisposition to bipolar disorder exists in our family genes so there is a constant fear and anxiety I have about its future surfacing in the family. I am making every effort to reconcile that fear and control it as it is important to understand that there are many worse ailments humans can have.

I am still perplexed if bipolar disorder is hereditary, or if it is partly environmental. I was told by a doctor once that you can delay the onset, but if the gene is there, it's there and will surface at some point by usually age twenty-six. There are mixed studies and data on this however. Environment can contribute to the onset but the mystery to me is that does it just delay the inevitable onset if it's a stable environment for children and then they are in the clear by their mid-twenties or can late life stress trigger the gene and land them into the disorder even at say age fifty? I would love to be certain, for my own children's sake. I would love to have that peace of mind that there is an age line that if you pass it, the worry plagues you no more.

    I recall being told by a medical expert if one parent is bipolar and the other is not and has no family history of it, then there is a 10 percent chance your children may have it. If both parents are bipolar, I believe the percentage is 25 percent, but I'm no medical expert. The percentages could differ in actuality – but that's how I recall them now years later after pregnancy and having originally posed the question to the doctor. With my second child, I was categorized as high risk due to bipolar disorder and took medicines that during pregnancy were considered to be in the safe class of drugs but nonetheless needed to be monitored. They titrated down my antipsychotic drug during pregnancy, and two weeks prior to pregnancy they removed it completely so the baby's liver would metabolize on its own, they told me. This is where I learned about the percentage chance of passing this disorder on to my children. Those percentages are branded into my memory forever with unease.

    I always pray that my loved ones come through fine in life and have happiness, health, longevity, success, prosperity, and good moral character with a soul mate of their own to be with them through their lifetime. I am hopeful that the stability we can continually provide the kids will allow this disorder not to be triggered in them. I would love to be reassured that if our children have stability, security and care in their environment then maybe it will never trigger an otherwise dormant bipolar gene. I hope that bipolar disorder if only exacerbated by environment hopefully will manifest itself earlier in life at such a time in life when I as a parent am still able bodied enough to help intervene in the rodeo I've weathered through myself. But part of me also wonders can you suppress the gene entirely from manifesting itself if you maintain a stable environment throughout your lifetime. Emilia and Delilah never became manic, but I did. I contemplate at times whether it was environmental stressors or genetics or a mix that triggered the manifestation of bipolar disorder type I in me. My sisters' lives were difficult in many ways as well. They never had a manic side and they both can go days without proper sleep without it triggering any mania in them.

I write this book to help others like me and to be a memoir for my children. My children in their teens now still don't know about their mom's bipolar illness and that, God forbid, might be carried forward in genetics. Keeping a dairy gives one closure. I am happy that I have written such a dairy – it has helped me. This book has given me clarity and closure to a past life that seems riddled with failures and mistakes.

I hope sufferers can find a sound medical professional that comes to understand them well and is able to help them through their journey. I am fortunate to have found a competent psychiatrist who I currently have been in the care of for many years. Not all psychiatrists are created equal. They have to significantly up their game to deal with someone who is high functioning, someone who can mask their episode in a half hour consultation, and in general has a lot of medical questions. I inquire about what-if scenarios to plan for all future possibilities I can anticipate. My current psychiatrist is excellent. She is irreplaceable to me. My previous psychiatrists were comparatively lethargic in manner with me.

My current psychiatrist has really blown it out of the water for me, prescribing aggressive sleep medicines as a remedy to deflect a manic episode and explaining how each is to be used and in what combination. She explains and quantifies the time frame of correction based on known medical averages. Aside from mental health questions; she nailed a physical ailment with ease that my family doctor was perplexed by. I told her I was craving dirt for quite some time. My family physician was stunted and just said not to do it, that dirt was unhealthy and I could get sick. I stared at her as that didn't really help the 'why' of the situation. But my current psychiatrist immediately said,

"Check your iron level. The craving for dirt is called pica. You might have very low iron" Indeed it turned out that my iron was direly low when the results came back, low to an almost anemic level. I immediately went on liquid iron supplements and corrected it. My psychiatrist was also the first to realize I had taken a particular antipsychotic for twenty years, which could build prolactin levels that could then cause brain tumors. My prolactin, when tested, was at 120; I think that was six times higher than normal for women. She switched me to another medicine in that same class of anti-psychotic drugs, which took my usual nine to ten hours of required sleep and grogginess in the morning away and replaced it with seven to eight hours of refreshing sleep that I awoke from much easier.

One of my cousins suspected with bipolar disorder died of a brain aneurism in his twenties. The family said that was the cause of death. But there were rumors it might have been suicide. Him and I used to play video games together. He was very difficult, like me. His dad had hit him a lot. His sisters were never reprimanded by his dad, their mom was in-charge of the daughters' disciplining. My cousin was the only one afflicted with bipolar disorder in his immediate family. His mother did have a temper. But it was hidden from all if she had bipolar disorder. My cousin was clinically depressed when Grandma Edna died. He left to go to another province in his teen years, as he had a falling out with family and worked at a gas station as his livelihood – living with a host family in the extended clan. He remained estranged from his family for a decade before returning to them in his mid twenties. A few years thereafter he died suddenly.

How I wish he and I could have talked directly at least once on having bipolar disorder. But the stigma was there. No one wanted to bring it up or speculate out in the open even within the extended family. These formal barriers existed. Too much embarrassment and insecurity over the illness drifted in the air.

One of my guiding lights through my illness was remembering what my dad said when my diagnosis happened in my teen years. Dad told me Prime Minister Winston Churchill led his country through World War II. He had bipolar disorder. Dad said if Churchill could do that even with this illness then I certainly could make it in life too.

I never considered myself downtrodden again just because I had bipolar. I wasn't going to fall into the self pity trap. I monitored myself incessantly. I self corrected upticks in behavior and set up checks and balances as much as possible. I also never put on horrendous weight because of the medicines which was a common side effect to these. It helped greatly that I weighed daily, charted and was very self-aware. I reminded myself to look at those above my achievement, not below. For it is an easy trap to lower the expectations for yourself if you look at those you have been able to easily surpass. I tried to stay far from self-pity, although that deep pit is enticing to give into and one where you stay oblivious to owning any issues in its betraying comfort. Silently I felt Dad had not owned his illness in the season of life when we needed him most, and I couldn't make the same mistake.

Sometimes bipolar disorder patients swing like a pendulum, with what is called rapid cycling. There must be an ideal medicinal balance for everyone and hopefully it's caught earlier in one's life. But even though you are on medicines when stressful life events occur either exciting or saddening, I have to compensate with additional medicinal adjustments so that I can remain stable. Just being on medication itself is not a guarantee of staying episode free. Continuous monitoring and adjustments are critical.

I need medicine management at this point, not counseling, not a psychologist, just a psychiatrist who can prescribe medicines. I need to stay accountable to myself and others to stay on my medicines so that I can be a functioning citizen and treat people as I want to be treated myself.

Going back to the issue of weight, a favorite topic in America, it can be a very difficult issue with those of us taking psychiatric medicines where some of these affect your appetite and often in the less desirable direction. My doctor mentioned to me I've done an uncharacteristically amazing job of keeping my weight steady even after medication switches over the years. I attribute this success to always being aware of where the measurements and weight sit on a weekly and sometimes daily basis. I have kept a running log of weight in a spreadsheet for seven years, and add to it daily, or most days anyways. My weight hasn't fluctuated more than five pounds in the five years I worked from home. Many colleagues struggled with weight upon working from home. But I managed okay in the home environment. In contrast the rough year working outside the house last year landed me 12 extra pounds – I could not find time to keep up with the log or weighing myself consistently every morning during that year. I've dropped ten of those pounds finally but still working on getting back to where I was at. This weight gain wasn't medicinally driven but rather lifestyle and stress related. It's a continual battle on maintaining your weight as you age. As soon as I give up the battle and am content with my weight is when the happy weight starts to pile on. We get complacent quickly if we relax our weight standards as we age. I cannot eat like I did when I was 35. I certainly cannot eat like I did when I was 30. It gets harder every year to maintain the weight you are at. The classic saying goes this way: 'It will never be as easy to lose weight as it is now'. The older one get the harder it gets, every passing year. Disciplined diet and exercise become so integral with age. Conditioning the physical form is so important to maintain focus mentally as well. I find the importance of exercise grows especially with age, keeping acuity and mindfulness. Exercise is therapeutic in ways and healthy for the mind. And food will always be there, I should not rush in all at once ever.

The self-awareness of a disorder and conquering it and saying you are bigger than that illness is so critical to recognize. I am not bipolar. I have bipolar disorder. Bipolar isn't my identity. I've kept from telling friends as I don't want them to assume instability where there is none. I worry they may jump to conclusions like: "She's super happy" or "She's super sad" and "Might it be a bipolar thing?"

I've reached the inflexion point in my life where I consider not hiding it anymore; there's no good in feeding into a social stigma. Many of us in the population are suffering in silence, alone with our mental health issues. It is more damaging to keep oneself so solitary with the knowledge eating away at us.

This is a biological illness; there is a chemical imbalance in the bipolar brain. Just like diabetes is a chemical imbalance of insulin in the body.

Why am I judged so harshly and made fun of? Why do people casually say, "The weather is bipolar today" or "The teacher is laughing like she's bipolar." Don't do that; don't use the word like that. It makes us wince. It makes us try not to look away. It makes us feel ashamed. It makes us realize you have no idea what this illness is about.

There were times in life where I regret not getting the counseling for certain life events in my childhood. One of these times where I wish I had worked out the monsters in my brain sooner was when Maddy was born. I hadn't worked out my own childhood incest issues in my head. I feared for my daughter. I had this anxiety when I looked at her in Darrell's lap or Darrell's dad's lap. Years later I told my husband of my ill-founded fear. Darrell was shocked and angry but tried not to express the anger. He didn't understand but just asked pointedly, "You've got it worked out in your head now, right? That there is nothing to worry about?"

I said yes, but I reflected inside myself that it is conditioned behavior from my fears in childhood.

It was new to me, men who didn't hit or men that were not angled towards perversion. I hadn't seen very many men who respected women and girls while I grew up in the Indo-Canadian community. I had seen men who mainly valued boys. It was very much a patriarchal Indian society in our 'Little India' suburb of

Vancouver. During high school, us Indian girls would be frustrated and beside ourselves commiserating to one another how the boys at home got their own cars when they turned sixteen and only had to do the infrequent outside chores, but the girls had to be confined inside, not be out late like their brothers, and do all the daily indoor domestic chores.

My husband was very much about equal gender roles for kids, where both will do dishes and both will mow the lawn. And I figured, too, that the gender segregation of duties will fall into place naturally as the kids get older, when it's easier for Hudson to mow the lawn and Maddy to do the gardening.

Out of necessity I mowed the lawn in my teen years, on a curvy hilly backyard and front yard with a mower that was set too low and was not self propelled. There wasn't a guy around to do it, and Delilah was about 20 pounds lighter than me, and Emilia was too young. My back hurt at night the day I mowed. Flipping the mower over to get the old oil out of it and put new oil in at the beginning of each season was rough. I'm sure there was another way to drain the oil but I didn't know how to. I didn't know much about mowers. I was definitely the outlier being a girl that mowed a lawn. It made me proud of myself though to a degree. It was grinding hard work but against the grain of Indian life. Most all else conformed with the patriarchal life and standards in our Little India. Emilia was very much at odds with Indian societal standards as she grew older and even more fiercely independent than Delilah and I. Emilia had less patience for gender inequalities that Delilah and I would hate as well but we differed in that we didn't vocalize much and went with the flow. Emilia grew up detesting everything Indian.

My mom handled each of her daughters very differently based on their personalities. Mom always, without hesitation, got into my older sister Delilah's space but Delilah never displayed that she minded it much. Mom would tell her matter-of-factly not to do this or that and without explanation, and Mom would get openly frustrated with her even in Delilah's adulthood. With me she was more timid. I was far away, and we had had three years of a hiatus during my first episode after Maddy, and then I was headstrong in general. I was my own person now, grown up. My values aren't my mom's values; and my mom's value's aren't mine. It took some adjustment, but she respects that.

I feel my mom and I have had our ups and downs together but the journey behind us on managing this illness together has been one where she is my continual rock, like Darrell. Both of these people in my life know when the onset of slight hypomania takes over, they understand the difference between good excitement and hypo-manic excitement. I am thankful for loved ones in my life I connect with daily. I call my mom very frequently, even for a few minutes we always try to touch base daily. She can tell by my voice if I am worried, mad, happy, or feeling down. She also recognizes the difference between episodic emotion and what is just genuine everyday happy or sad behavior. I used to feel abrasive if she and Darrell spoke about my mood, but for many years now I've matured in that regard. It doesn't bother me anymore; I know they are a type of check and balance for me. I cringe at the thought of not having them in my life. I hope we all have someone to lean on. I hope we all have someone who will recognize when there is an imbalance starting to happen and get help for us. Equally important is for one to be fully accepting of their vulnerability to the illness and be open-minded to receive help. There is a tendency to get defensive and in mania especially the grandiosity makes you feel like you are the only wise one and everyone else is far inferior; there is also a strong tendency to dismiss other's concerns and deny there is an issue.

I feel like I've transcended this boundary where I am not in denial that the issue is with me. I've tried continually training my mind for open acceptance of the fact that I can easily regress into bipolar disorder phases without being fully aware and I need to trust loved individuals around me to tell me the right thing to do and not take their intervention as insulting. I am hoping I've built the habit of self awareness, continuous self monitoring, and also the habit of not to become defensive and create a barrier of denial that I need help. I constantly remind myself of my regrettable actions when manic in the past and that is usually enough to force me to remain cognizant and open to feedback from loved ones if I am climbing an upswing and Darrel or mom make me aware of the elevated behavior.

On the subject of denial, my little sister is another story – although not born with bipolar disorder or any manic tendencies she has been perpetually fighting depression for the past decade. Emilia has always felt that she isn't treated like an adult by her family. She feels Indian standards are such that by now she was to be married and attain the status of a mother which would afford her greater autonomy from her own mother and meddling aunts. My mom has been awfully careful in recent years not to place societal expectations on her. Living back under one roof for mom and Emilia was difficult. Emilia's untreated depression for the first few months was an issue feeding into her continual negativity and comments. Her humor is often dark and condescending in nature. Emilia wasn't on medicines and was feeling down. No one really realized that she may need a medicinal regimen on a permanent basis. My husband would ask me, "Are you sure she doesn't have bipolar disorder as well?" That's when I researched and found that Dysthymia (Persistent Depressive Disorder) was a diagnosis and for life. I wonder if Emilia can be helped with this knowledge. She hasn't talked to me in many months and is often defensive on any issue. Mom can tell Delilah anything in terms of a reprimand, I've become significantly calm like Delilah towards Mom over the years as well, but Emilia gets to the point of being argumentatively defensive with even the slightest feedback given to her by family. I wonder if some of it is not in her control. She has had a difficult life of her own. Acclimating back to living with mom has been an adjustment for her. We worry for her depressive state and trying to find the rhyme or reason to when the downturn creeps in. The persistence of it makes me wonder about this disorder.

The following sheds some light on Persistent Depressive Disorder:

For a diagnosis of persistent depressive disorder, the main indication for an adult differs somewhat from that of a child:

- *For an adult, depressed mood occurs most of the day for two or more years*
- *For a child, depressed mood or irritability occurs most of the day for at least one year*

Symptoms caused by persistent depressive disorder can vary from person to person. When persistent depressive disorder starts before age 21, it's called early onset; if it starts at age 21 or older, it's called late onset.
— www.mayoclinic.org

Related to Emilia, in response to Darrell's query on her possibly having bipolar disorder, I said, "No, she's never manic. She can go on without sleep for a while."

Emilia has never been manic, so I researched further, and I think it's clinical depression for life, known as Dysthymia. I told my mom about this possibility and how we might help her stay on medicines. I sent Mom a medical link to her phone about the disorder and it was poor timing as Emilia happened to see it and she was offended. I feel she'll be able to lead a fuller life and find her inner happiness and balance if she is open to figuring out whether there is an imbalance that needs to be corrected. In Canada it used to be hard to get a referral to a psychiatrist, I'm not sure the situation now but I hope she finds the ideal medicinal balance. When I went through my first set of medicines back in high school it was trial and error. Now it seems more scientific a process; in the US I've heard the medical field does a heavy amount of blood tests and monitoring for weeks to get one to the closest ideal set of their medicines. Quality and thoroughness of care can differ depending on your loved one's knowledge of resources and finding the right expert provider, support groups and sometimes good health insurance impacts the level of care.

My mom is now in her sixties and set in her ways. Emilia was on her own for twelve years. To co-live now, even in a larger house, is frustrating to divide responsibilities. But thankfully this past month, Emilia has come out of her depression and is involved with Delilah's kids. Emilia is the cool aunt to the teen kids and dotes on the younger two who are only eleven months apart. I earnestly pray for my little sister to have happiness, peace, and contentment in life.

My doctor says luckily for my family I'm not a violent person. That's very hard for a family, to help that person and manage their own safety when violence is involved. Like the situation with Dad, I don't think we threw in the towel too early as it couldn't be salvaged due to the violence. Mental health providers typically ask the question of new patients: Do you have a gun at home? They ask for various reasons – both suicidal and if a threat to others.

I grew up in tumultuous conditions. Life is stable now. I'm thankful for what I have and harbor an odd anxiety looking to the future but hope that this illness will never trouble me again. I modify that prayer at times to acknowledge life will happen again, but give me the perseverance to manage it better. There may be a time when illness hits, and I don't have a supportive spouse around anymore in old age. Or what if the apocalypse happens, and I have no more medicines stockpiled and have to fend for my kids in a horrible world? I did stockpile this medicine when they said the world might end in 2012 and at which time I asked my seasoned psychiatrist if I could make these substances out of nature if I had to. She said flatly no, they are made in a lab.

For me at this stage, there was somewhat relief with the last couple episodes; they were milder and recovery was quicker. I owe it to a large base of medicines I now know how to use. My doctor has a level of trust in my judgment when I'm not in an episode. But when one is coming on, I call her or email and tell her I'm going to adjust my antipsychotic medicine dose upward. I copy my husband on the emails too and she feels more confident that a loved one who is caring for me has weighed in as well. You don't know when judgment will slip from you. It's easy to fake being coherent and stable in a short consultation with a doctor. The loved ones who have seen you for a while know your norm versus an episodic persona. They need to talk to the doctor and at the time you feel they are the bad guy for doing so. I was angry at Mom and Darrell at times for talking with the doctors. I thought they were judging me in a sinister way, it was the irritable symptom in me. Only later when non-episodic you realize, wait, it's okay. They were crying out of concern and hiding it and trying to keep it together when talking to the doctor. Don't be mean. Understand what you are putting them through.

I have a longstanding regret about lying to my husband about my illness. My husband's and my relationship was built on a lie when we got engaged, from the onset. Even though Dr. Singh, while I was in college, had warned me firmly, "Any life partner you choose, you make sure you tell them about your illness first before becoming committed."

I said "Of course" picturing a loving marriage where I could be open about this. I regret not telling my husband about this. In reality when you meet someone you really take a liking to and want to spend the rest of your life with – sometimes a fear creeps in that they might leave you if you tell them. You fear it may jeopardize the whole relationship. That was my decision when I met Darrell, that I would hide it until he loved me and wouldn't leave. I didn't want to sabotage my chances with him.

My mom kept pushing me. "We need to tell Bethany, to be sure they are okay with it. It is important to be honest in this relationship Alayna!" But Aunt Jennifer and I convinced my mom not to say anything to Bethany. We figured I was fine, no need to say anything and risk nullification of the arrangement. Aunt Jennifer and I feared they might rescind the proposal.

That fall once I got engaged and after I'd spent a week visiting Darrell's sister with him at her house... I felt his gentle kindness. I really felt at that moment I wanted to tell him everything but I waited until I saw my mom to see if I should. She was angered. She said, "No, it's too late. This was supposed to be shared beforehand. It would seem like trickery to share it now. Suck it up and stay fine the rest of your life."

I had to make sure I had a job and could afford my own medicine. I'd tell Darrell they were vitamins, and he was indeed confused the first time he had to go pick them up from the pharmacy, but he was so unobtrusive about it. He didn't ask any questions that first year. He didn't know what was coming. My first episode he'd ever see was after I had Maddy, during the postpartum period. And that was the scariest and most severe one for him during our married life. He had not been given any education on this illness or warning – I should have told him about the illness so he wasn't entirely blindsided.

Darrell's parents were somewhat resentful that I had hidden my illness, especially blaming my mom; she should have known better. They were resentful I had *hidden* the fact that I had bipolar, not resentful that I was *born* bipolar. I tried explaining to them that it was me, but they said Lydia should have overridden my decision. She was the adult who was to make that decision, I was only 22 when the proposal was made. They just didn't know how best to manage the illness. Bethany had told me years later, we would have been ready to handle it then and prepared had we known from the onset, and that we would have been appeased by the honesty in the pre-engagement phase.

I had so much anger and hate toward the memories of my childhood that after that 2006 episode, I didn't talk to Mom for three years. My husband was also mad that she hadn't called to give him the heads-up about what bad shape his wife was flying back in from Vancouver, fully manic with an infant daughter in her arms. Or a call for him to fly there as a support for a wife that is falling apart.

I continued dialogue with my sisters during those three years. Mom once talked to me during that period. "Maybe you should seek counseling for what happened during childhood" She had said gently. I was angry all over again with her. But I am ashamed of that time, that I didn't talk to her all those years.

I understand Mom's life now. As a mom, myself – I understand how hard it is to rear children and parents can't be expected to be perfect.

I was hurting though during those years. But Mom luckily was at peace during this time only because she knew I was in touch with my sisters and that all was okay with me. That was enough for her. She had had several large surgeries during those three years, which makes me even more upset with myself for why I hadn't reached once or reconciled with her sooner.

It makes me sick with myself. Mom had gone through so much pain all her life – physically and emotionally. The last visit landed me in an episode that shook up my world, my marriage, and aged my mother- and father-in-law considerably. I can't go back, ever, I had thought in those years. As my children grew older and I faced parental exhaustion and challenges the appreciation of all Mom had done came in like a tidal wave. I had Darrell to lean on for support, she had had no one.

My almost high school aged children wonder what they want to be. Maybe medical, maybe investment banking. They throw it around but it's still too early to decide.

I worry about their stress level when they reach their early adulthood. I fear they might have my ailment, and it's my earnest prayer that they don't have what I have. But they do have a mom and dad who are educated on the illness. Other parents are hit with this whirlwind of unknowns on how to handle this. I pray my kids will like psychiatry. Mental illness is on the rise. Perhaps it's better diagnosed now and thus on the rise, or the technologically tilted generation is plagued with greater anxiety. The devices are creating more issues for its patrons that are glued to a lit up screen all day – Children and adults manage their social media accounts and try to keep at bay their feeling of FOMO and depression. Mental illness has never been more of an issue and the minds are becoming more fragile it seems, perhaps debilitating by this growing technology use and dependence. Many feel their existence is validated by only the number of likes and followers on their social media accounts and anxiety creeps in quickly if their friends don't text them back within a few seconds.

My kids hopefully won't need to help their mom in her older years with her illness; I have my repertoire of medicines and especially sleep ones that regulate me. At least I hope I can keep it together the rest of my life and not burden them. But Maddy and Hudson would be amazing healers, as they can get in the mind of their mom one day. Becoming a therapist could be draining. I hear even therapists now have a mandatory rule to see a therapist. But being a psychiatrist may not drain them as much; medicinal management and an assessment of highs and lows and prescription writing might work for them and not overly stress them. As soon as counseling is sought by a patient a psychiatrist typically will deflect the flow of discussion and refer to the appropriate level of expert in the psychiatric field. I wonder if my children will be interested in this healing field. I think they would have a real time case study in front of them always.

My psychiatrist and I have long conversations and often go over the appointment time limit when time allows and there is no next patient if it's the last appointment of the day. She says she enjoys talking to me and can talk to me for days. It makes me feel good about myself. It's a deep dive into a very self aware bipolar brain for her continual assessment.

I hope dearly that the stigma of mental illness goes away. So many times I've wanted to be honest with my bosses. I have bipolar disorder. Help me and understand me. I can do good work, but I'll have my occasional ups and downs that I need time to resituate through.

The secrecy makes me cry. Only my family and Marina know; they are the only ones I can tell so far. Besides immediate family some in the extended family had heard I went to the hospital. The circle of knowledge on my illness has been very small. The reason for this is that the bipolar disorder becomes your overriding identity to those not bonded with you. Family is family; friends can be transient. You only meet a handful of friends in your life whom you can truly trust. But circumstances and things change. What does not change is bloodlines. There hopefully is a level of loyalty there that doesn't falter as easily as friendships do.

I've stopped praying for a cure to bipolar disorder. I can lead a pretty good life still even with the illness. On the surface of it most of my life I am unencumbered by the illness. Unlike in the case of diabetes that follows one daily and even hourly. Diabetes is a high maintenance illness where I would need to prick my finger for blood to test my levels daily, and sometimes strap on an insulin button infuser that auto-feeds medicine into the side of my body throughout the day. I also should be thankful I don't have cancer, or some other severe ailment that is also permanent like bipolar disorder or that is terminal. Bipolar disorder has this unnecessary shadow of stigma and the unfortunate upkeep for daily secrecy is there. Secrecy from friends, neighbors, coworkers, etc. In the current society we live in it feels that way – like it needs to be kept confidential into perpetuity. You cannot easily share the burden of it like the way a diabetic, cancer, or heart patient can share their burden openly.

I wish there were greater openness even within the extended family. With my paternal grandfather and my father having bipolar disorder, and with thirty grandkids on the paternal side, there are likely more of us even in my generation. Delilah and I have our guesses on who might have it in addition to me, but it's so stigmatized and no word of it beyond our secretive discussions. I hope society moves forward. I don't know if some of my aunts would fly off the handle if I approached them and said I have this, I struggle with this, tell me about your situation. I'd like to help and share my experiences. But there maybe radio silence, extreme offense taken, and subjects changed quickly. I don't know which way the pendulum would swing. So we stay quiet, pretend it's not there, and continue on.

With increased mental health issues surfacing and the staggering statistic of every one in five now afflicted with an illness at some point in life, we need this openness now more than ever. As a world society, we need to understand the stranger sitting on the subway crying and speaking to Jesus is just like one of us, but the flashes in that person's brain are going quicker than normal. The missing lithium is triggering what onlookers might interpret as an obtuse character.

With bipolar disorder I notice my latent energy when a stay at home mom at times creeps up and there is a driving need to be ultra productive. I need to use this bubble of productive energy, so in the past I had filed a utility patent on a children's wall art slide piece I made. I had this exciting pent up creativity to me I had to use and apply. But when it came to pursue the prototype the costs were prohibitive. I later learned that additional energy daily should be focused on a consistent sustained productive habit that can keep my focus. I see the commercials for manic episode medication and the lady that is vigorously painting the house with that wide eyed look reminds me of my overly productive energy at times when there isn't much to apply myself to. There doesn't seem to be a happy medium if you aren't constantly applying yourself, either you'll swing into depression or go into mania. Routine is key and forming habits to do roughly at the same time every day helps consistency of mind.

As the well known '80 20 Rule' goes … Twenty percent of life is what happens to you, and eighty percent is how you handle it. You can lead a full life, even with bipolar disorder, it is your self acceptance, support system planning and awareness that will help harness this challenge.

I wish I had given up audit and tax and general accounting long ago and pursued something else I like that was engaging to me; my circumstances financially had allowed that flexibility. I just never let go or recognized that liberty; especially after my green card made that possible to stop the employment status. I am not sure a kid ever grows up dreaming he or she wants to become an accountant. It is the practical thing to do at some point simply. I had considered being a lawyer while growing up but that would be an added three extra years of law school on top of a bachelors degree, so added costs and I my paramount consideration was to get out and earn after four years of college to alleviate my single mom's burden.

I was climbing a slippery corporate ladder and was barely at the third rung. I'm glad there is more work-life balance and work from home now for me. Am I excited about numbers and accounting? Not really, it was the commonsensical approach to get through college and make money when I graduated twenty years ago. Now I wonder what I really want to do with the remaining twenty five years of my working career. I continue the contract gig for now. I can accommodate my illness better while working from home. Candidly speaking numbers don't excite me. That might sound sacrilegious to say as a CPA. They never really did. Conversely it is the people that excite me, and I look forward to utilizing my accounting experience with a people facing career like business development in accounting and finance or a CPA recruiting role.

I once overheard a conversation at the Multinational CPA firm in the east coast town decades ago; it was a disturbing one where my fellow auditors were making fun of someone who had come in during the audit fieldwork in the morning to a client office in another state and it was reported he had been shaking nervously and suddenly had said his doctor told him this job wasn't good for him. After this outburst he had abruptly left the conference room. They had laughed; but in my mind's eye I saw this individual, and pictured him with pressured speech, trying to convey his thoughts but they were coming out in an unfocused manner. Here my colleagues were laughing at this young man they didn't know personally, about how he exclaimed the job wasn't for him and he had abruptly left the company – like some sort of freak. The other audit seniors were chuckling at the story told to them by their counterpart, all the while their comedic tone suggested they purely felt this guy was a loser and lightweight for handling his job. But I immediately understood, it was another person like me struggling to maintain mental stability.

We suffer in silence and unnecessarily so. I want to find other people with bipolar disorder like me. I often look around in my circles and wonder, one percent of all the people I know have what I have. Worldwide 2.4% have bipolar disorder. .

Who are you? Can we talk? I am approachable. See me, hear me. We can cry together, laugh together, and look into each other's eyes for that silent understanding only another person with bipolar disorder has, of similar fears and anxieties. Maybe one day society will evolve forward, and the mental health stigma will end. We'll just be known as a different kind of "diabetic" patient.

Humans only use 20 percent of their brains. In mania I wonder if we end up using more than that. They say if humans used 90–100 percent of their brain capacity, what wonders would be possible? Telepathy? Could we move things with the powers of our mind? Maybe bipolar disorder has some genius aspect to it, if harnessed at the right time and left in some perfect balance of early hypomania.

Shakespeare and Einstein had bipolar disorder. I don't know how stable their home life was other than it was alleged that Shakespeare had abandoned his family. Sadly, both geniuses were likely untreated cases. We didn't have chemical labs formulating medicines that could bring mania down back then. But Shakespeare and Einstein may not have left society the gifts they did had mania not crept in. Bipolar disorder looks different from person to person. This manic energy is a frightening power, but if harnessed at the right time with self-awareness maintained, you can take advantage of it. Attention Deficit Hyperactivity Disorder (ADHD) I read is now considered a form of genius. Perhaps bipolar disorder has already demonstrated its positive contributions to society by such geniuses. Could their rare level of genius have been made possible to them due to their chemical brain imbalance?

There is an optimal balance of hypomania. On ascending that manic curve up its left side there is an area above the normal line where productivity peaks. I've built an illustration of this below:

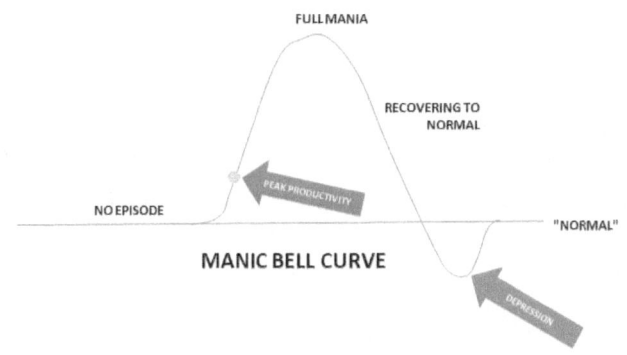

There is this area on the manic bell curve graph where the arrow on the left notes "PEAK PRODUCTIVITY." You are not yet at full hyper-mania at that point. The ideal circumstance I hypothesize is to stay there for a bit but then come back down or have the medicines in place to not allow you continue the climb. I say "normal" in quotations in the diagram; everyone has a different normal. Some personalities are just high strung. It's not the bipolar disorder. It's the person and their attributes they are born with and developed along the way due to their life interactions. But mania has its own acute symptoms that can be differentiated and diagnosed with its unique characteristics of lack of focus and the patient not standing still with one topic and instead jumping to the next completely unrelated topic without ever coming back to the original subject matter.

One can have coherent and enhanced creativity at this high-productivity stage and, depending on your profession, as a scientist or a writer, if you continue to ascend that curve, you might have some genius break through ideas. I am curious where on the spectrum of the curve Shakespeare was when he wrote down his unsurpassed masterpieces.

My Dad would explain to me that the flashes in the brain between poles increase from the standard of fifty per second to five thousand every second. I'm not sure if that's at all factually accurate, but in theory, I get it. One has sped up their flickering faster, in mania, where your words come out too fast, and your thoughts race. You are processing at a pace too fast for coherence when these flashes are at their peak and your mania remains untreated. You've had no sedation injection or heavy medicines to treat your mania and push it downwards. You exhibit pressured speech, you talk a mile a minute. The chart in the first part of the book scaling the depression to mania spectrum shows a detailed account of symptoms on each level of the bipolar pendulum. In addition to this chart in the first chapter, this graph shows the progression and regression when one enters and exits through an episode.

This 'peak productivity' area is fascinating and amazing in certain ways – it is part of the onset of the first stages of mania, called hypomania. This is the phase at that ideal part of the bell curve which creates the brain power like you've never seen before. It creates the magnetic personality, charisma, enhanced confidence, and articulate speech. I speculate the following two possibilities during this stage of hypomania that lends the enhanced abilities:

The chemistry in my brain is as such that I'm using much more of a percentage of my brain than the standard human does which is approximated at no more than 10 percent on average.

Or

The chemistry in my brain is causing the processing of information to go faster than normal and there's an ideal speed before the flashes go too fast, within that ideal speed there is a peak in creativity and productive capacities while still remaining coherent.

These two possibilities are what I hypothesize could cause an enhanced creative capacity and interpretation speed.

How did Einstein and Shakespeare attain their breakthroughs? Was it their bipolar minds that allowed creative genius? It could possibly be that their gifts to society were made possible by their bipolar trait which comes at a high price to these individuals.

In ancient times individuals suffering from bipolar disorder were classified as deeply unstable people who were markedly erratic. There were stories that some would stay in groups up in the mountains or wilderness only to come down to the village and cry profusely in their depression. Such accounts were kept in various historic diaries over the centuries. On the polar opposite end these same individuals would be in euphoria and theatrical for the villagers amusement, perhaps it depended on the season and amount of sunlight to dictate what pattern of behavior they exhibited. I remember once Mom told us girls that Dad's moods might be correlated with the seasons as she noticed an exacerbation during those change over times. In ancient times these mysterious swings in mood likely were attributed to the person's character, not a disease.

I'm thankful for the era I was born in and that my life may not be as short and neglected as those ancient individuals suffering from the same illness as I have. I'm also deeply thankful for medicines which after trial and error I have arrived at a chemically balanced medium for my age, weight, and biology.

Mania can be embarrassing – those ancient people may have felt embarrassed in the aftermath and thus hid in the woods most of the year only until their imbalance made them seek the village again. But you aren't aware of that embarrassment until afterwards when judgment returns weeks or months later. In this age things like social media and email create a digital footprint that makes some of those manic actions permanent for all to see years later. Blunders shared with others many times over, not just erased from the on-lookers memories overtime. This digital footprint era maybe more enlightened but also just as much precarious to creating permanently marked reputations.

It's a medical fact: people with bipolar disorder live shorter lives. Maybe it's due to damaged relationships, work or school performance stress, depression implications or the side effects of anti-psychotic medicines. Below is a release in 2014 on this area of longevity and bipolar disorder:

The average reduction in life expectancy in people with bipolar disorder is between nine and 20 years, while it is 10 to 20 years for schizophrenia, between nine and 24 years for drug and alcohol abuse, and around seven to 11 years for recurrent depression. The loss of years among heavy smokers is eight to 10 years.
— www.sciencedaily.com

You might continue to ascend the manic curve and inevitably fall from its peak. Or you may remain in the depression of that sinusoidal curve that typically continues its ups and downs during many bipolar disorder patients' lives. For those hit more with depression, I read somewhere that it naturally can go away on it's without treatment. But then there is the permanent depression that I spoke of that I suspect Emilia has. There is also the risk of suicide if untreated.

On this matter of depression duration:

On average, an episode of major depression lasts 4 to 8 months, although this duration can be shortened by treatment. Most people recover within 3 to 6 months with treatment, although it can take longer than this for some.
— www.mydr.com.au

To shake off depression naturally and biologically without medicines is a tough feat, and for your loved ones to weather it and be always vigilant night and day on suicide watch erodes part of their life too.

There is a heavily taxing patience needed and sometimes this runs out for loved ones. I make an effort to show my loved ones appreciation while I can and am in my own.

Life is too short, even shorter for us with bipolar disorder. One must reflect on where on the medical spectrum mental illness is compared to many other illness types that plague one tenfold worse. There are more challenging health issues than bipolar disorder that plague an individual's body. Bipolar disorder plagues your soul, your mind. It is an illness where your mind becomes your biggest enemy. The mind is the most dangerous thing during an episode. But there are worse things that are less controllable even with a support system.

I've learned I cannot consider myself infallible based on my past experiences and cannot take comfort in the fact that my episodes are becoming less severe with age. There is no rest assuredness that the remainder of my life will never become unstable again or imbalanced. My self-awareness may not protect me from another episode. It likely will need to be a combination of loved ones intervening and a pre-setup support system. You could elect to have a conservator for legal purposes even as an adult, as one can burn through assets completely unchecked in an episode. I have to keep in mind even hypomania, not full mania, can be damaging to relationships and circumstances. One can burn many bridges during a manic episode that cannot be rebuilt later. I keep an open mind that I am not invincible to this ailment, ever. I can have a series of checks and balances in place; a greater degree of openness with those outside immediate family to watch for signs in me. If I lack that circle long term I will need to see a mental health professional regularly who can accurately gauge the mood in a longer conversation and give guidance on medicinal adjustments. I may need to check myself into a hospital. To be rendered clueless and fully episodic happens all the time to individuals. It is a scary journey alone if with only the transient company of strangers alongside you sporadically who may see you as just high strung and extremely extroverted and not give the behavior a second thought. A stranger is unlikely to intervene, there is no vested relationship. A friend or family member has the frequency of interaction – they may recognize that hidden fire erupting in the brain.

Individuals with bipolar disorder have a more delicate chemical balance in the brain that needs to rebalance, simply put. We need to drop the stigma of this illness in our society. Look around you. One in every one hundred is suffering in the US, and it might not just be bipolar disorder. There are a multitude of mental health illnesses that uptick this ratio in the population to 20%, or one in five people. They should call them physical brain illnesses instead of 'mental' ones.

I don't judge homeless people anymore. They were put there because of some childhood trauma or abuse or neglect or mental illness their family or foster care could no longer tolerate.

I cringe that my dad ended up in soup kitchens at times. So did a bipolar actress in Hollywood I remember it being reported by her on a national TV documentary when she was blindsided by a bout of depression that came on and she had wandered aimlessly for days.

I pray for a stigma-free world. I pray to find others like me, just one other person I know who has bipolar disorder that I can talk to. Tears come to my eyes when I write this. In my forty years, I haven't known a single one willing to speak openly about it, other than those I bumped into years ago at the psychiatric ward that were open to talking about it. I had taken some phone numbers down while there. Those numbers were lost, no one ever called me either, and so we never kept in touch. My doctor at that time had even dissuaded me from contacting one of them as that patient was struggling with suicidal tendencies still.

Many people suffer from loneliness and a person with bipolar disorder even more so. My philosophy is to smile understandingly at people in the subway and don't look away if they look unhappy or unstable. The power of a smile can change a lot for a person. It releases your endorphins when you smile, and it releases theirs too. It could make their day, or possibly even reverse a decision of harm they were going to make.

I often recall a story of a man who was mentally unstable on the subway. He didn't have weapons or a gun, and everyone was avoiding him and trying to flee to the next boxcar over or get off on the next stop. Everyone was trying not to make eye contact. Another brave man pulled him into an embrace, and the deranged gentleman stopped his yelling and cried and cried on this stranger's shoulder, until help came.

The power of that hug perhaps saved someone from a suicide later. That's the kind of humanity I pray replicates itself in our cold, fast-paced, technological, and unfortunately weapon filled world.

I believe technology is desensitizing children who grow up as mass shooters in the loneliness and the overwhelming feeling of a lack of belonging in a world rampant with cyber-bullying. A world where bullying doesn't stay at school like it used to but rather follows you 24 hours / 7 days a week / 365 days a year on social media.

Everyone has a story. I myself should consider putting my personal device down more often and smiling at those people who need that smile; a smile that could change a life. Maybe I'll find another person that way, who has bipolar disorder like me. Even thinking about how wonderful that would be, I shake uncontrollably with tears of joy running down my face as the loneliness of suffering it alone will end.

I've been a high-functioning bipolar patient who never went to group counseling. I never wanted to uncover the truth that I had this illness. It would tank my career to put myself out there I thought, and then I reassure myself I'm pretty solid otherwise. I need medication management, not so much counseling or group therapy. However I suffer alone, and a support group would help.

I still live with the constant fear of the next life event that might trigger an episode. Like a parent passing away, God forbid. I have no bipolar support network that is also high functioning. I don't think a support group of professionals with bipolar exists. They'd keep it hidden, they'd never say it out loud. They'd risk losing credibility if their client base knew they had a mental illness. Unfortunately that is the current reality of the perspective in this world today – eclipsed by stigma.

So we continue to suffer alone. Hidden. Silent. We continue to pretend we don't have bipolar disorder. But there is hope, through advocacy like the National Alliance of Mental Illness and such programs I read about recently, we can continue to build awareness, eradicate the stigma, and foster acceptance of mental illnesses. After all it affects 20% of the world's population. No longer should such a majority hide in silence.

Being able to write my life down in these pages has been a healing process. We live in a culture that is still very secretive about mental illness. Today my reliable cohort is my husband and my mom. They are integral to my stability factor and they can anticipate my illness. The journey behind me makes me realize this illness is not just about medicines but a trusted circle of loved ones. I hope each of us can build our trusted circle and broaden it ever so widely.

Afterword

Suicide is an irreversible decision. While I've been fortunate to gain self awareness and generally stand on the manic end of the pendulum and not the depressed end – I have considered suicide during one post-manic episode where depression hit in its aftermath.

The ramp up of an episode, either to mania or depression, if intervened with early enough medicinally could help an individual greatly. As an episode progresses one loses the brain balance and the judgment is just not there to stop an irreversible decision from happening – like suicide. Early diagnosis and intervention is crucial.

The first step to having a plan is to not be in denial of one's illness. Understanding that one is susceptible and predisposed to certain outcomes is critical. Once a person goes down that slippery slope of not getting help and being in denial, the episode continues its ascension and judgment and decision making is greatly impaired. This first step of acceptance grows into the next possible step of being able to be self-aware. Consider telling your loved ones, like close family and friends what to watch for and ask them to make you aware of what they see if they find pressured speech and a jump from subject to subject without correlation on your end. It may be a symptom towards mania. Conversely look for a loss of interest in people and activities or a persistent sadness without cause, it maybe the onset of depression. The symptoms chart in Chapter One from www.bipolaruk.org is an insightful summary of what to watch for in loved ones or yourself.

Monitoring one's sleep patterns may help and learning your particular trigger or hallmark symptom is critical. Please don't delay the help; medicinally this mania or depression could be corrected. The quicker the intervention is made, the faster the recovery. There most always is a transition period to acclimate to new medication, even the best most suitable kind will yield some sleepiness or other side effects initially. These are bothersome but patience and perseverance will help one come out of it eventually as one acclimates to the new medicinal regimen.

Depression typically takes a long time to wear off on its own and can persist. You could make a permanent decision that doesn't bring you back from it. Be kind to yourself, formulate a written self rescue plan and share it with your trusted circle. The plan could encompass what they should watch for, when and what doctor to call, etc. Seek help from loved ones or a support group, you are not alone, ever – call for help. Please keep in mind the following resource:

National Suicide Prevention Lifeline
1-800-273-8255
Help is available
Speak with a counselor today

https://suicidepreventionlifeline.org

Additionally a vast peer led national support organization exists for two groups – both those directly suffering from mental illness and also the family members caring for the loved one dealing with the mental illness. There are local chapters throughout the US that offer support groups to alleviate the aloneness which both the family and individuals afflicted are burdened with and are otherwise journeying with this illness alone. This peer led support group organization has information at:

National Alliance on Mental Illness
www.nami.org

Also please know there are a multitude of support groups on social media that exist as a virtual forum for a vast network of thousands of members and active participators walking the same road – there are even more granular groups specifically for spouses and parents supporting a loved one with bipolar disorder. The supporting loved one's travel alongside this illness can be overshadowed by solitude but doesn't have to be. You quickly realize you are not alone in that vast world of virtual support groups where everyone has complete autonomy to be candid about their situations.

Many illnesses of the mind are simply a chemical imbalance and a trial and error process initially must be used to find the perfect combination of medicines for an individual; such medicines can be changed and doses adjusted later as your circumstances in life change. Acceptance, self awareness, and a network of support are what I hope people will be able to attain and keep on a sustained level during their lifetime. There are many of us dealing with the same challenges silently. We shouldn't have to travel this journey isolated and alone.

www.ingramcontent.com/pod-product-compliance
Lightning Source LLC
Chambersburg PA
CBHW020637220526
45464CB00001B/187